THE HUDDLE

An experience of hearing voices and living with other personalities

Janet E. Cooper

chipmunkapublishing
the mental health publisher
empowering people who hear voices

Janet Cooper

All rights reserved, no part of this publication may be reproduced by any means, electronic, mechanical photocopying, documentary, film or in any other format without prior written permission of the publisher.

>Published by
Chipmunkapublishing
PO Box 6872
Brentwood
Essex CM13 1ZT
United Kingdom

http://www.chipmunkapublishing.com

Copyright © Janet Cooper 2009

Edited by Catherine Garvin

Chipmunkapublishing gratefully acknowledge the support of Arts Council England.

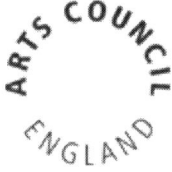

THE HUDDLE

Dedicated to Dr. Elinor Kapp, Consultant
Psychiatrist, without whose help and expertise,
patience and love, I would not be alive.
She was wise beyond her profession!
Thanks Elinor! – and remember not to hurry!!
God bless you!

Janet Cooper

THE HUDDLE

AUTHOR'S NOTE

I wrote this book in 1996 when I was very depressed. At the time it proved wonderfully therapeutic and cathartic, even though the battle to get through each chapter was tormentingly real and profoundly challenging. Today, 26th February 2008, I signed the contract for its publication.

This book explains how I started hearing voices at the age of fourteen and the various ways I coped, or didn't cope, as the case may be. I describe very vividly what it's like to hear voices and what they say. It is a very raw account, peppered with both humour and self pity! Always there is the real me struggling to find some way through.

I recount my positive therapy with a Consultant Psychiatrist following a disastrous and dangerous exorcism attempt by a Baptist Minister, which landed me in a psychiatric hospital. I struggled out of this man's harsh theology to discover, among the same scriptures he had used against me, a healing and very precious relationship with the Son of the God I had once hated. From darkness to light, from hate to love, from pain to healing………

Rachel, one of my other personalities has also written her story which I have included towards the end of this volume. She gives an incredible, detailed account of the exorcisms we both endured, followed by a chapter outlining her love for the Jesus she was repeatedly told hated her. Also included are a few examples of music we wrote to help cope with the voices. I suppose it all adds up to a pretty unique account!!

Janet Cooper

This is a psychiatric journey, a spiritual journey, often a depressing and repeatedly morbid journey, but also a human journey. A tormented soul somehow hanging on in there until a light gets switched on.

In fact, many lights were switched on along the way and I did eventually stop hearing voices. That is, I stopped hearing The Huddle. From then on there was no holding me back! I went to Cardiff University where I studied Theology, graduating in 2001 with a first class honours degree and clutching a prize for the highest exam marks, excelling in biblical languages Greek and Hebrew. I was accepted to study for a Masters degree, but due to being unable to fund further studies I went to work for Lloyds TSB in the hope of saving my tuition fees. I worked in their contact centre at Duffryn, Newport, for four years, actually getting paid to hear voices!

Unfortunately I became very unwell. I underwent several major abdominal surgeries, following a mistake made during an emergency hysterectomy procedure, for which I was awarded medical negligence compensation. No amount of money can, however, compensate for the fact that I am left in constant pain, unable to work, I now walk with a slight limp, and, perhaps the cruellest blow of all, The Huddle came back!

After eight years of being Huddle free, I have them back. But different! They are different! It had taken me lots of effort to learn to live *without* them, now I have to learn to live *with* them all over again. The reasons for their return, and explanations of why and how they are different, I intend to tackle in

THE HUDDLE

my next book. This book remains largely as it was written twelve years ago.

Please, come with me on this part of my journey…….

Janet Cooper

THE HUDDLE

INTRODUCTION

Silence!

I have, for a long time now, nurtured the idea of writing a book about The Huddle, and fantasised over the final outcome of such a project. The fantasy being, that when I have finished, when I have written the very last word, The Huddle will be gone, catharsis complete, and written upon the very last page would be one glorious, wonderful, triumphant word,

SILENCE!!!

Silence is something I do not have because I am a voice hearer. I hear voices. Sometimes I wonder what other people are hearing when they do not hear these sort of voices. Is there silence or are there other noises? What *is* silence exactly? I understand it only as an absence of The Huddle.

I don't want this book to be an account, or an attempt at an explanation, of *why* I hear voices – although an element of exploring that issue may become inevitable – but rather an account of the fact that I *do* hear them. What is it like? How do I live with them? How do I cope?

Notice that I write about hearing these voices as fact. I do not *think* that I hear them; they are not loud thoughts, or hallucinations, or memories of people. They are real. Real and separate voices. I can hear them as surely as I can hear the voice of another person in the same room. So how do I sort out whether I'm hearing one of my voices, or a human being? Easy peasy! Like, if you have your radio on, people talking on it, and somebody walks up and speaks to you, even without seeing that somebody you'd know the difference. Also, my voices are nearly always plural and I know what they sound like. They are easily recognisable to me just as the voices of people I know are easily recognizable. I am used to my voices, and besides which, it would be impossible for a human being to speak to me or about me in the loud, vitriolic manner that The Huddle use. At least I like to believe it would be!

So. I recognise The Huddle. No problem about that. I call my voices 'The Huddle' because they are just that. A Huddle. A group huddled together. Sometimes I think that 'The Huddle' is too friendly a title for them, but that is what I refer to them as, and that is what they are and shall remain. The Huddle.

I do not want to go into my life history in any more detail than is necessary for the writing of this account. Neither, initially, did I want to discuss any aspect of my multiple personality, but after much thought I realise that it might just be a tad impossible to write a book about hearing voices without including details of my other persona.

At the time of writing I am aware of five other, younger, personalities who live alongside me. I am careful not to seek out any others who might be lurking about in my head and am also determined that my mind shall 'create' no others to live with me, with us. At times it is difficult to think of *myself* – singular – and the effort to keep up reference to 'I' and 'me' and 'my' is constant and exhausting. I

THE HUDDLE

shall endeavour to keep the writing of this account as *my* own work. I shall be 'I'.

Maybe my fantasy is a ridiculous hope! – that by writing about The Huddle I shall somehow work them out of my system, or at least come to a greater understanding about what is happening to me and an increased ability to cope with my miserable situation. I want to encourage myself as I write. I want to prove to myself that I can cope, and am coping. I want this project to be yet another positive coping mechanism.

What I do not want to do as I write, is to find myself plunging the depths of some wretched, useless self pity for page after page, although some wallowing may be inevitable. Weak creature that I am!

So let's get on with it! A book about the Huddle! Where on earth do I begin? Was there ever a clearly defined beginning to all this?

Not sure!

So write!!.................

Janet Cooper

THE HUDDLE

1. In the beginning.
2. Others and an Angel.
3. Demons?
4. A Lonely and Secret Malady.
5. Feeling a Bit Angry!
6. Food for The Huddle.
7. My Psychiatrist and other Coping Strategies.
8. Drugs.
9. Christmas 1996.
10. Marriage and The Huddle.
11. What of the future?

Janet Cooper

THE HUDDLE

CHAPTER ONE   IN THE BEGINNING

I was fourteen years old when I first started to hear voices in my head. Or was I? Did I hear them before then? Did I have 'good' voices that didn't bother me at all? I don't know, so I shall write instead that I was fourteen years of age when I first heard a *nasty* voice inside my head. I remember that day as if it was yesterday – it is still crystal clear to me although obviously not as disturbing as it was twenty five years ago! The nasty voices started in school like this.....

My history teacher had always made it abundantly clear that she didn't like me and the feeling was certainly mutual. She insisted on calling me always by my surname whilst calling the other lasses in my class by their first names. That wasn't nice and I not only disliked this woman, I hated her guts, and every history lesson was an utter misery for me. Because of her attitude towards me I would either deliberately make no effort at all in the subject or else go all out to be good at it in the hope of impressing her and getting into her good books. She frequently made me so angry that I would be determined to prove to her that I wasn't as stupid as she thought I was! I never succeeded: Even a degree in history at the age of fourteen would not have impressed her where I was concerned!

Anyway, on this particular day, a Friday, my class had a history test. 'Hitler's Rise to Power.' I remember that so well, and as I had learned my work thoroughly I was not in the least bit worried about writing my essay. It would be a doddle, and I was confident of obtaining a reasonable, if not good, result. I'd show the stupid, ridiculous woman! The silly cow…….

It was time for the test to begin. I wrote my name at the top of the first sheet of writing paper, but as I went to begin writing my first sentence I heard someone calling my name. Loudly, suddenly, urgently. A male voice. I was startled and turned quickly to look around the classroom to see who it was and what they wanted, calling out to me like that. Everybody was scribbling away, however, and appeared not to have heard this voice. Was I the only one? How puzzling, and not a little scary! My pulse began to beat a frantic tattoo on my chest wall as I went to put pen to paper again, only to be interrupted.

"Don't write anything! You can't write!" This was authoritative and commanding. It went on, even more insistently, "Don't you dare write one word on that sheet of paper!" And so I didn't. Every effort I made to begin my essay was greeted by this voice telling me not to write. The words, 'or else', seemed to hang in the air, unspoken, but as a very real threat.

I glanced around several times during the thirty minute duration of the test and saw that everyone else was busy writing away, heads bent over desks, oblivious to whoever was yelling at me. Mrs. History Ma'am invigilated, pacing slowly back and forth at the front of the classroom and thankfully not looking over any shoulders to see what was being written! Her eyes remained fixed on the floor as if she was looking for something she'd dropped. It

THE HUDDLE

occurred to me that nobody had heard this voice but me.

Other sounds bombarded my ears and seemed extra loud. The interruptions to the silence of the classroom made by the occasional cough, the dropping of a pen, a fidget, the rustle of paper, a thoughtful sniff..... The room smelled strongly of leather satchels and floor polish. Time ticked on and still I wrote nothing. I was startled, scared and confused. I didn't know what to do or how to react. So I sat there, bent over my desk, pen in hand, pretending to be busy and hoping nobody would notice I wasn't writing.

Mrs. History Ma'am was furious when she collected my empty sheets of paper. She was probably secretly delighted as well because she then had a valid excuse to have a go at me and show me up in front of the rest of the class.

She took the sheet of paper bearing only my name and held it out at arm's length. She then turned it over, peering at it closely, as if she had missed something, opening her eyes wider, scratching her head, looking for the writing that wasn't there. She was being very dramatic about it and everyone started to laugh. Everyone, that is, except me.

"Bishop? A word if you please! Now either my eyesight needs testing or else you are using a pen with invisible ink!" The laughter increased. "Where, if I may be as bold as to ask, is your answer?" I couldn't open my mouth, never mind give her a reply. "Well? I'm waiting with great interest Bishop!"

The laughter stopped abruptly as she raised her voice to me and set her face before me, eyes blazing. My then silent classmates sat at their desks, motionless, looking appropriately pained and serious as they waited for the fun to continue.

"Somebody told me not to write anything, Miss." I eventually managed to say.

Oh! I see! Somebody told you not to write anything, did they? I don't think I've heard *that* one before!" She paused here for effect. Boy, was she enjoying this, the rotten cow! "And who exactly *is* this somebody who told you not to write anything? Maybe I should have a word in their ear before they go around telling everyone else not to write anything."

"I don't know Miss." I replied rather pathetically, but truthfully. My voice shook and silent tears rolled down each cheek in an unchecked torrent. Mrs. History Ma'am ignored my watery distress and continued to enjoy herself.

"Well, just you listen to me *Miss Bishop*! Nobody, but nobody, ever does this in one of *my* history tests! DO YOU HEAR ME?? How *dare* you not do the set revision! How *dare* you! Well, there's somebody telling you to write something now, Miss Bishop, and that somebody is me, and I am telling you that I want one thousand lines from you by the time this weekend is over. One thousand! Did you hear that? One thousand. 'I must learn my work for a history test'. One thousand times, and don't think I won't be counting them. And heaven help you girl if they are not in my hand on Monday morning! DO YOU UNDERSTAND??"

THE HUDDLE

Sobbing and unable to speak, I nodded my head. It wasn't my fault! I *had* done my revision! I knew more about Hitler's rise to power than flaming Hitler would have known! It wasn't fair. Gee, I hated that woman!

There had been a horrified, audible gasp from the rest of the class as my punishment was doled out. Fifty lines. One hundred lines. Even two hundred lines. Fine. Okay. But *one thousand*? Nobody was ever given one thousand lines! I was inundated with advice on what to do and friendly pats on the back as soon as Mrs. History Ma'am had stormed out of the classroom and we could no longer hear the quick click, click, click of her high heels along the corridor. But the other kids weren't *really* comforting me. They had secretly enjoyed what had happened and showing relief, gloating, and being glad that it hadn't happened to them! It's so easy to appear to be sympathetic about something when that something hasn't happened to you, isn't it?

Many years later, a Baptist minister's wife said this to me,

"Yes, well, right, but you see Janet, if that had happened to me I would not have taken any notice. I would most surely have known it was wrong to sit there and write nothing. That's how I am, you see. I *do* know that I would not have obeyed a voice like that!" Whilst she was saying this to me, I had sat and cried over my foolish weakness. Now I can feel very angry about her cruel words and think, well, bully for you, Mrs. Clever Clogs! Glad you had such strength of character! How easy for you now to sit there and say that you wouldn't have taken the slightest scrap of notice when a voice nobody else could hear suddenly started yelling at you and scared you half witless! But then it never happened to you, did it, so how the hell can you say how you would have reacted? Silly mare!

Back to the day of the history test. At home that evening I plucked up the courage to tell my Dad that I'd been given one thousand lines because I hadn't given an answer to a history test. I didn't tell him *why* I'd not written anything – can't remember if he even asked me why. Dad was puzzled at my apparent lack of revision, but also annoyed at the severity of the punishment inflicted, and it was years later that my mother told me how he'd written to the headmaster complaining about it and Mr. Martin had written back that I need not have done all those lines! However, at the time my father insisted that I write them and so I gritted my teeth and set about my task that very evening.

I had the whole weekend ahead of me and no way was I planning to spend it writing lines! However, one thousand lines take a lot of writing and I quickly realised that most of my weekend would have to be spent writing one sentence over and over again. My fear, bewilderment and misery soon gave way to anger, bitterness and hatred. I really wanted to 'get back' at that rotten, unreasonable teacher. So I spoke inside my head to the voice I'd heard, and found that I could get a reply! It would converse with me! Wow! I knew it wasn't 'nice' talk, but I didn't mind what it was saying, the way I was feeling. It was talking about

THE HUDDLE

Mrs. History Ma'am and what I could do to get my own back on her. I could hate her and curse her and damn her to Hell! So I did! Inside my head, gleefully, I hated her and cursed her and damned her to Hell! It felt so good to do it and I wished she would drop dead on the spot! Mrs. History Ma'am!

The following Monday she was not in school, so I did not have the sweet pleasure of telling her that my father was sending my lines to the headmaster. I did feel genuinely surprised and guilty to learn that Mrs. History Ma'am had, in fact, been rushed into hospital that weekend and would be off school for several weeks. I was also genuinely delighted and thrilled, and so was the voice in my head!

Over the next few weeks I began to hear more voices. A group of them. A huddle of them. Sometimes they would all talk at the same time, rather like being in a crowded room yet still a little separate from it all. Often, one or two voices would come out of this group and talk to me and I discovered that they knew what I was thinking, and I could talk back to them in 'think' language inside my head. I was most aware of this happening when I wasn't busy or concentrating on anything in particular. Sometimes they were nice to me, commenting favourably on anything I was doing, but they quickly became critical and obscene. Their swearing was awful, and, like they still do, they would call me names – a slut, a stupid bloody idiot, a fat, ugly cow, etc.. They always told me that they hated me, and put me down at every opportunity. Still do. Day after day after day after day...... Little wonder that I continue to dislike myself and have a rock bottom self esteem.

Back then I would have done almost anything to get The Huddle to like me, but I no longer seemed to be able to control my own mind. Where did these voices come from, anyway? Who were they? What were they? Did everyone else have voices in their heads?

Then one day during that perplexing period, I heard someone say to someone else during the course of a conversation,

"A little voice told me...." Now I believe that was a misquote of that well known and used phrase, 'a little bird told me', but all those years ago I thought, that's it! Other people were the same as me! Other people had voices too! I wasn't any different at all. Well thank goodness for that!

By then the voices were warning me not to tell anyone about them. Or else. It was to be our own special secret. Or else. They would reward me for keeping it and punish me if I didn't. They told me I was special because I had them, and so I started doing the silly things they told me to do. Like scratching my body with pins and scissors, pricking my fingers and squeezing out some blood to smear in a cross upon my forehead. Like sitting in front of a mirror and..... I came to believe that something terrible would happen, such as my parents dropping dead, if I disobeyed the voices or else told about my secrets.

So there we are. The history test I tend to think of as the start of my hearing voices experiences. But then one day not so long ago I was talking to my psychiatrist, Dr. Kapp, about the five imaginary friends I had when I was a little girl. Their names were Agnes, Ingrid, Yolanda, Maria and Zena. I

THE HUDDLE

found myself telling Dr. Kapp how these friends had always been around for me, helping me, liking me, and only ever saying nice things to me. *Saying.* I described them as if they had talked to me. Had they? Or had they only spoken as part of my imagination, in 'thought' language?

I told Dr. Kapp how these five friends used to watch me as I played the piano. They would stand on the stairs in a close group (huddled) and look at me through the open sitting room door, from where they would discuss how clever I was, how nicely I played and how pretty I was. They said the things about me that nobody else did, and therefore I didn't believe. Still don't! They came to school with me; they watched over me, they slept in my bedroom with me. A group, huddle, of five young girls with plaits like I had. I liked them. I needed them. It was as the bad voices took hold that these wonderful friends who said all the nice stuff gradually faded from my mind. But had everything about them been pure imagination? Or had I really been hearing them as voices? That would mean that I'd been a voice hearer from the time I was a very small child and might explain why I never complained to anyone about the bad voices. I maybe accepted them so readily simply because I was already used to hearing voices in my head. It was just the way I happened to be. It's the way I am now. Maybe nice friends became nasty friends. Nice voices became nasty voices. But why?

It's hard to answer that question, so all I will say now is that, at fourteen, stressful things had happened and were happening, and I was a very withdrawn, deeply unhappy teenager. Maybe it was my depressive state which brought about this 'bad voices' state. Chuck in a few teenage hormones and WOMPH!! It did not occur to me at the time that it was wrong or different to hear these voices and I didn't consider it as something I needed to complain to somebody about. Years later I discussed this with my mother. She informed me that my G.P. had told her I had 'psychological problems' and then proceeded to do absolutely nothing about them! I was a highly neurotic, shy, awkward, severely withdrawn teenager who would grow out of it.

But I didn't grow out of it! I coped with it. What choice did I have? I somehow muddled unhappily through the years, got married at eighteen, had the first of my two beautiful children eight years later, and continued to be profoundly unhappy. I don't want to go into detail about those years because this is not supposed to be my life story, just an account of The Huddle, but some background is obviously necessary.

They had not been easy years. I suffered terrible and prolonged depressions and many psychosomatic illnesses. I went through violent mood swings and my husband, Frank, found me difficult to live with. (He wasn't exactly Mr. Easy Peasy himself mind!) Our twenty years of marriage owes much credit to his patience and love towards me – and mine towards him!! So many times during the early years of our marriage he would yell at me,

"You need a bloody psychiatrist!" Yes. He was right, although I didn't know it or believe it at that time. I did not think there was anything at all wrong with me!

THE HUDDLE

The voices had, by then, become particularly blasphemous and, along with them, I was viciously against anything to do with God. Frank hid his Bible as I stormed through the house, looking for it, threatening to rip it to shreds. He recalls that I appeared to be different people at different times, a sort of Jekyll and Hyde. At times I would become vague and go into a trancelike state that was difficult to snap me out of. Other times I'd storm out of the house, usually at night, and wander the streets, not knowing why or where I was going. On my return home I would not be able to remember where I'd been. I know now that I'd probably been under the influence of one of my other personalities, probably Rachel. Frequent thoughts of suicide were encouraged by the voices who would, and still do, chant,

"Kill yourself, kill yourself, kill yourself, kill yourself……."

What a miserable and tiresome way to live.

My children, my son and my daughter, were very young when I was offered hope and shown the light at the end of my tunnel after I confided in a church minister about my terrible depressions. As we talked, Reverend H. went on to ask me if I ever heard voices. I replied in the affirmative and told him a bit about them, despite the warnings in my head to shut the f**k up! (It must have been one of my stronger days!)

Over the next two years I ended up telling Reverend H. almost everything about the voices and now bitterly regret that. He was neither a psychiatrist nor a skilled counsellor and I was to become very ill and distressed whilst under his care. It was also an unnecessary nightmare for my family who suffered through it all with me.

Reverend H. told me that due to a previous deep involvement in the occult these voices were demons that had possessed me and I needed to be delivered from them, and he was God's chosen delivery man. He would command them to go after I'd confessed and repented of all my sins and asked Jesus into my heart. Simple as that! They would go and I would be free. How easy it sounded. Oh! That it had been that simple and that easy!!

In my depressed and highly vulnerable state I believed this man, and hope was indeed kindled within me. I found myself more than willing to go along with him and do exactly as he said, especially as both he and Mrs. H. seemed willing to spend so much time and effort to see that I was delivered. It turned out to be a false and soul shattering hope, and the interest these people showed in my plight I now see as voyeuristic curiosity, Mr. H. barely concealing his pride in having authority over my life and my 'demons', and hoping his church would be mightily blessed by God when such a sinner was eventually delivered!! What followed was a long and extremely traumatic attempt at exorcism which I am still struggling to deal with and recover from. My then newly found faith and trust in God was torn to shreds, my personality more firmly established itself as multiple, and my marriage was very nearly destroyed.

I continued to become worse and worse all the time Rev. and Mrs. H. were 'dealing' with me. The

THE HUDDLE

voices at times were unbearable and I was sure I would go stark, staring mad. I spent two short spells in St. Cadoc's Psychiatric Hospital which didn't prove helpful as I believed all they wanted to do was drug me up and lock me away. At the end of my tether one cold March day, thinking things could get no worse, I drove to a lonely spot, wanting to escape, be alone, think, kill myself …… but I wasn't alone. I was raped. I thought he was going to steal my car when he came towards me, and hadn't expected to be grappled to the floor, my head clunked, a vicious knee bruised my thigh, then out of this world terror as he……

Looking back now, that attack probably saved my life because afterwards I became so wrapped up in trying to deny, and cope with, what had happened to me that I lost the urgent, overwhelming desire to carry out what I'd desperately wanted to do. Kill myself. I was frantic about going to the police, thinking (because you read this sort of thing in the news etc.) that they wouldn't believe me, or they'd blame me for being where I was. But the police at Maindee Station in Newport were wonderful and couldn't have been more helpful. Most importantly as far as this book is concerned, they put me in touch with Dr. Kapp, the psychiatrist I still see on a regular basis. She was used by them to counsel victims of sexual abuse.

It was about five months after I was raped that Dr. Kapp visited me for the first time. I was curled up on my settee that afternoon, absolutely terrified and dreading her visit. Frank answered her knock on the door and as soon as she walked into my living-room I took one look at her and thought, 'Oh no! This isn't going to work!' She reminded me of an over strict school ma'am, but I quickly learned not to judge this book by its cover, as she was not like that at all. Within minutes my greatest concern, that she would be like a female version of Reverend H., was dispelled, as she was nothing like him whatsoever. Phew!! She spoke softly. Quietly. She didn't touch me, grab me or shout at me. She was not out to judge me, condemn me, lecture me or tell me I was a category 'A' sinner. She was to become somebody I could trust (almost!) and somebody with whom I felt safe, and I needed someone to feel safe with….

It remains a long and painful journey. There have been tears and despair and anger and hatred. At times I've felt like hating Dr. Kapp as she has nudged me gently, and sometimes not too gently, along the road of psychotherapy. There has also been joy and laughter and much love as she has come to know and accept me exactly as I am at any one time. (And vice versa!!) She has never treated me as if I have some dreadful illness or 'condition'; rather she has guided me along the path to wholeness and the healing of my mind. Not because I'm ill. Or possessed! But because I have been damaged. That's the way I like to think of it anyway.

It is not wrong to hear voices. It is just different. It is also at times a complete and utter misery. At this very moment, as I am typing this, The Huddle are grouped together in the lamp on my desk. Guess what they are telling me? They are telling me, ordering me, not to write, but I am far enough along the road now to ignore their ridiculous

THE HUDDLE

instructions. It's not always so easy though, and at times I do still give in to them. They hate the fact that I'm writing a book about them, or at least attempting to! I wonder if they will allow me to finish it!?

Let battle commence!!

Janet Cooper

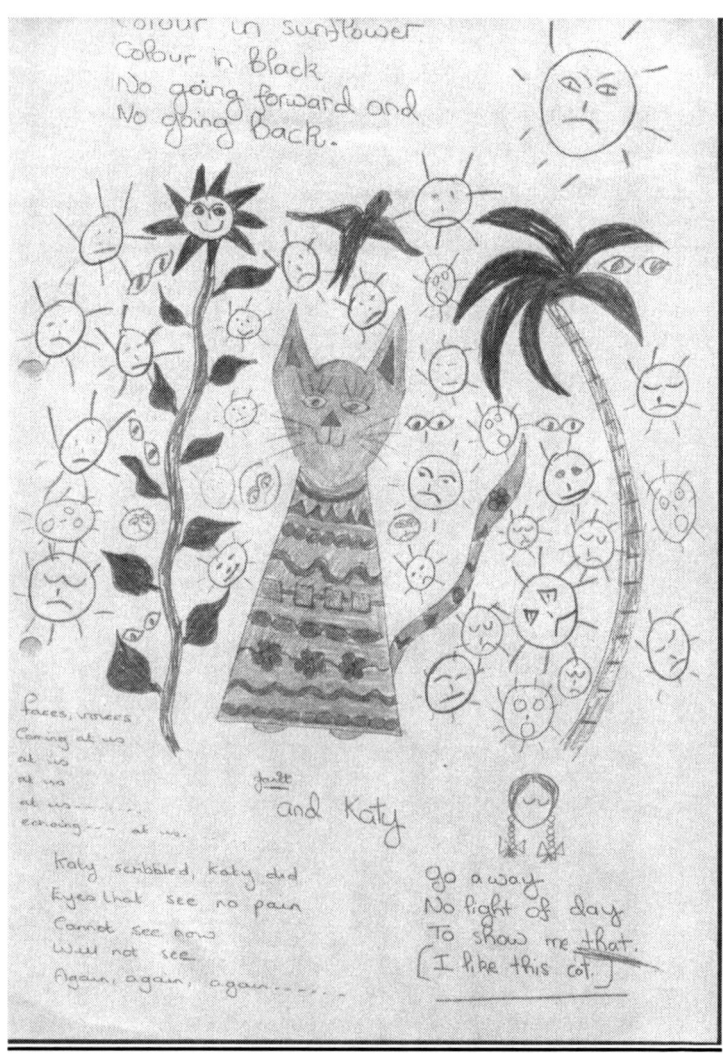

THE HUDDLE

CHAPTER TWO   OTHERS AND AN ANGEL

So there we are. The Huddle is a group of voices that I hear. They are always a group. Always huddled together. Always a Huddle. But now I am going to explain about two other, entirely separate voices that I also hear. One of them is Rachel. The other one is called Angel.

I wrote about having five other personalities. Maybe now is a good time to introduce them to you. (Or should that be you to them?) I'll begin by listing their names and ages. First of all is Jan, who I believe keeps up with me chronologically. Then there is Rachel, 17. Liz, 16. Katy, 12, and little Janny who is 3. I remind myself of a Russian doll! Dolls that get smaller and smaller until you reach the perfect little baby in the middle. The one that can't be broken apart. Layers of dolls like layers of personalities. Is there a perfect little person in the middle of me who can't be broken apart?

Rachel is the one that I have real contact with. We are able to speak to each other, hold conversations, discussions and, frequently, arguments. I hear Rachel as a voice in my right ear. She lives inside my head in a bare, grey cell built from breeze blocks and she refuses to decorate her cell to make it pretty. I don't know why. She has a window through which she can see out when she wants to, and curtains to pull across when she wants to be alone and away from the world. She is able to listen in on my life and frequently does so, knowing near enough everything about me. Rachel is also able to 'come out' and use my body; she's written many letters to Dr. Kapp and even posted them, all done without my knowing. I've only known about these letters when Dr. Kapp herself tells me about them. Scary. Rachel will tease me by saying that she has written dozens of letters telling Dr. Kapp the most awful things about me and what a thoroughly obnoxious piece of work I am. Charming! Yet charming she is not!!

Rachel also likes to help around the house and is particularly fond of making beds. She delights in the fact that she makes them differently to how I make them, and it drives me wild to go upstairs to make the beds, only to find it had already been done, and not the way I like it done! It may sound petty, but it's frustrating and unsettling. I often 'lose' a couple of hours each day when Rachel is 'out'. This causes arguments between us and thus our relationship is, at best, a stormy one. Dr. Kapp has brought Rachel and I to the point where we no longer seriously hate each others guts, but there is still a lack of trust and a mutual dislike.

Now, while I am writing this, Rachel is profoundly depressed and refusing to speak to me. Frank tells me that she hasn't spoken to him either for several weeks although last night she did inform him that she is not well. I know that her silence is not a good silence. It is a sad and despairing silence I find wearying to live alongside. I 'see' her lying on the floor of her cell, staring ahead at a blank wall, often crying. She is frightened of falling asleep because of vivid dreams and nightmares. She is also frightened of staying awake……

Rachel hears The Huddle as well. The same way I hear them? I really don't know. She will refer to them as 'voices', rather than calling them The

THE HUDDLE

Huddle. I think what has happened to her over the past few weeks is that their constant abuse has finally overwhelmed her and she has simply given up fighting and coping and being strong. She used to be so strong, the strong one, stronger than me, but is now worn out by it all and is depressed and lethargic and hopeless.

I call to her inside my head. "Rachel?" but these days the only reply I get is "No! Go away! Leave me alone!" I am very worried about her and frightened that she will do something silly. She recently wrote an essay about herself that was so sad. "I live behind the face of someone but I am someone else…….."

Rachel is a little bit bigger than I am and has short, dark hair. I once drew a picture of her.

I don't talk to Jan, Liz, Katy or Janny and I'm not hearing them as voices at the moment. I am aware of them in many ways but unsure how aware of me they are. Rachel talks to Liz and Katy but mostly chooses not to because she says they upset her, get on her nerves, and she is not the slightest bit interested in anything they have to say anyway. So there! Dr. Kapp has spoken to the younger ones but I don't know if she's ever met Jan. Certainly Rachel, Liz and Katy have written to Dr. Kapp and drawn her pictures. Their writing is different from mine. Rachel writes with an untidy, hurried looking scrawl. Liz, oddly, only ever writes with her left hand, even though she is right handed, and so her script is somewhat squiggly. Katy has a neat, looped, twelve year old hand. Jan, I know, prints very neatly, and I myself have fairly small, neat writing.

Earlier this year Katy evidenced herself by repeatedly slashing me with a knife. She cut my arms, my back, my leg and my chest, leaving me looking as if I'd been clawed by a wild animal. It darn well felt like it! Thankfully Dr. Kapp was able to speak to her and talk her through it to the point where I've now not been cut for several months. That is such a relief! Apparently Katy had been thinking that I was like a man who'd once hurt her, and was coming back to attack her again, and so she was lashing out with the ensuing painful results. I'd been back and forth to my G.P. for stitches and steri-strips as some of the cuts had been deep. Dr. Sami was wonderfully patient towards me throughout all this and would often do the stitching himself rather than send me to the local hospital which I hated. The staff there were not exactly sympathetic and understanding and I always left the place in floods of tears.

Katy lives inside my head in a rather nice little bedroom, with a cosy bed which she sits on and a pretty rug on the floor. Katy screams a lot. I am aware of this even though I mostly cannot hear it like Rachel can. Katy was also once blind. An hysterical blindness because she was afraid that if she could see then she would see something very bad and evil which would hurt her. After getting to know and trust Dr. Kapp, Katy was able to see for brief periods and now, as far as I know, is able to see normally.

Liz is the personality I am least aware of. I know that she is sixteen and has long hair. She has

THE HUDDLE

recently taken to 'coming out' when I am in the kitchen, when she will indulge in being downright naughty – that's my best description. I will 'come back' into myself to find that a saucepan has burned dry, whatever was in it ruined, whereupon I was blaming Rachel who would viciously have a go at me for this false accusation. Then one day, out of the blue, Liz confessed to Dr. Kapp that she was responsible for the burned saucepans. But why? Liz was unable to give a reason for her behaviour and we all decided that she must have been doing it to attract attention. It made me so very fearful about what else Liz might do without me knowing. I am frequently anxious, scared and upset. "Shame!" snipe The Huddle!

Janny, little Janny, is the personality who, at present, distresses me the most. She does not seem to be aware of myself and the others in any way, but Rachel and I are certainly aware of her. Rachel hates having her around and becomes very upset when Janny is awake, so we are thankful that she sleeps for prolonged periods.

So how am I aware of little Janny? Well, I just feel very strongly that I have this little girl living inside me – it is a very real, almost physical sensation. I will sometimes do things that little girls do. I will hear childish words coming out of my mouth and find myself pointing to a toy, for example my daughter's bunny rabbit, and saying, "Rab rab! See rab rab? My rab rab!" When I feed the gerbils my mouth will speak, "There mouses, I like mouses!"

I lose time, become absent from myself, and then 'come round' sat on the floor playing with toys just as a small child would be playing. It is embarrassing and distressing when I can't control it. Thankfully, when I'm out of the house, I usually have my children with me, and hence an excuse for any childishness! Janny cries, and her crying, plus the other noises she makes, are pitiful and sad. Even not hearing her, I can feel it and sense it. She is a very sad and lonely little girl. Poor Janny!

I've deliberately left Jan until last as I don't want to write about her! I am jealous of her, she fascinates me, and I can't quite work her out. I am only ever aware of Jan when I am in work. I have a part time job which I believe I, as Janet, am incapable of carrying out because I am stupid and nobody likes me. So it is Jan who goes to work for me, enabling a necessary top-up to the household finances. When we arrive at work it is as if I take a few steps back out of my body and watch this Jan, so cool and calm, confidently carrying out her duties. She is extremely well liked, very good at her job, never swears, is cheerful and smiles easily. I wish I could be Jan!

So that's the briefest of introductions to the other persons in my head. I refuse to accept this as a 'disorder' because it is anything but disordered! Each person inside their own living space, with their own personality and their own autobiography. All extremely neat and ordered! A mind that is divided into people in order to preserve the whole. No disorder about that.

The very little I've read on the subject of Multiple Personality was written by an American guy who claimed to specialise in this 'disorder' (though as he didn't have it himself, I fail to see how he could be a

THE HUDDLE

specialist!!) He wrote about the afflicted persons having dozens and dozens of personalities, all popping up here and there to say hello! One of his clients had a personality who was a Red Indian Chief from hundreds of years ago, and another who was a burly lorry driver who loved to wear suspenders and bright red nail varnish! It all sounded pretty ridiculous and bizarre! I, as a 'we', am not ridiculous or bizarre, and very thankful I am not to be able to compete with these other tortured souls by producing dozens upon dozens of weird and wonderful alter egos. Another doctor wrote about his doubts that the condition even existed. Maybe because of the confusion inevitable when dealing with dozens and dozens of personalities. I'd like to meet that man and tell him that I do actually exist, albeit in the plural, and I am most certainly not a disorder! We are all many different people – I happen to manifest it in an exaggerated way. It is just the way I am, we are.

One dark and sleepless night I wrote a poem trying to describe myself.

Janet Cooper

ON BEING ME

Being Janet, me, is noisy, full of others and of them.
People live behind my face,
Voices shout and hate and whisper in my ears,
"You! Janet! – are a terrible disgrace!"
And worse.
And so much worse, so help me Lord.

In me, small people live in fear
Of what they know.
They never grow,
Just stay the same.
Not innocent and young
Like we all were the day this life begun.
I mean 'began', we get it wrong.
Past and present mixes up,
I am us, and then I get confused and curl up in a chair
To wish that I'm not here and never there.
So help me Lord.

And so I live with them inside my head.
A living Russian doll.
And yet I know them but I know them not!
Just that they're there –
A flash of memory, a hurting, a despair
Is all wrapped up in little people
That live inside my head.

I want to talk to Rachel, Katy, Liz…
The psychiatrist will say,

THE HUDDLE

And then that weird confusion
Just before I go away.
To where? To where?
Another person shall be there
To think and talk and cry.
I don't know where *I* go to,
It is her, then,
Never I.
So time has disappeared once more.
Psychiatrist gives a parting hug.
"Yes, I'm okay." I say, and shrug,
Pretending I don't want to ask, and say,
"I don't remember everything,
Who talked to you today then??"

The second voice I'm very aware of besides Rachel and The Huddle is that of an angel. Okay, okay, I know what you're thinking – I really must be cuckoo bananas and having religious hallucinations! But hang on a minute. If that sounds far fetched, crazy and ridiculous, then why? Is it any more ridiculous than having The Huddle and other people living inside my head? It was actually Rachel who kept insisting this voice was an angel; I'd simply been referring to it as a 'good' voice, as it says only good things and is never abusive and seeking my harm and destruction. In fact the opposite!

For example, I will often find myself in the kitchen, knife in hand, ready to cut myself because The Huddle keep telling me to do so and I get to the point of believing that if I give in to them and do as they say, then I will gain a few hours peace and quiet. I know that in reality it does not work out that way, but at times my resistance is rock bottom low. Why? Well, because The Huddle are capable of keeping on and on and on and on and on for hours and hours and hours and hours at a time about the same thing. When they have spent nearly all day chanting "Cut yourself, carve yourself, slash yourself in pieces, stupid bitch! Cut yourself, cut, cut, cut……do it, do it, now, now, now….." then it is sooooo tempting to obey them in the hope of shutting them up or at least getting them to change the subject. A change can seem as good as a rest some days. Anyway, in this sort of situation, Angel will often come to my rescue by her gentle suggestion, while the knife blade glints over my bared arm, "You don't need to do that, Janet." And so I don't do it. She can bring me to my senses and prevent any further harm. She shares my predicament on the spot, as it were, and I am then comforted and encouraged in my struggle to cope with The Huddle. Rachel wanted to call this good voice 'Angel' and so I finally gave in to her, giving the voice this name. Well, why not? A good voice in the midst of the obscene and blasphemous Huddle is indeed angelic and sweet to my mind. As far as I know, only Rachel and I can hear Angel.

We've only had Angel for about seven months. She arrived shortly after Dr. Kapp resumed my psychotherapy following a break. Dr. Kapp came back to find me dangerously suicidal, and were it not for her unexpected and well timed visit then I believe I would now be dead. So then I wouldn't have written this book, and you, dear reader, might well be doing something more useful than reading this! Anyway…

THE HUDDLE

We do not hear angel every day, and neither is it possible to hold a conversation with her. She simply makes short, sharp statements of encouragement and guidance. She appears, at all times, to be gentle and good and totally trustworthy. I went all poetic and wrote another poem. Yes, you've guessed, this one is about Angel.

I have an angel.
There is an angel in the dungeon of my mind
Who is lovely, good and kind.
She wanders through its chambers,
Through each room,
In which resides a tortured soul,
Despairing, dark, in gloom.

And angel sheds the light we fight against
For fear we'll like it
But it will not last.
And yet we secretly desire and pine
To in the sweet and lovely light recline
And live in peace.

We hear, I hear, foul demon voices
In whom the whole of hell rejoices
Just to do us harm.
Does Angel hear them too?
We do not know,
She will not say.

"Cease not to pray."
She whispers in my ear,
And we inside despair and cry.
Our prayerlessness is Satan's sly

Design to claim us still as his.
I want to kill me. I want to die!
"Please don't!"
Is Angel's gentle sigh.
And so I won't.

She says,
"The evil comforter has left.
You're sad, depressed, despairing and bereft.
But though you pine for him you left behind,
Cling now instead to me, to hope, to life,
Cling to the angel in the dungeon of your mind."

Aha! This poem has mentioned an evil comforter. My evil comforter. So who or what was my evil comforter? I don't suppose an explanation of this is particularly relevant to this account, but as this is my book then I can write what the hell I like in it! If I want to digress and ramble and waffle then I shall! So I will. Besides which, writing about my evil comforter will hopefully prove cathartic to the memory of. So here goes.....

At times I suffer from depression. I don't just get fed up and feel a bit down in the dumps. I get depressed. I have come to know the difference. Depression is a rock bottom pit of despair that you believe you are in forever. Black. Less than nothingness. Unbearable. It is hopeless, joyless, fruitless agony. Mental and physical torture. Nothing whatsoever worth living for. I fear and dread becoming depressed.

One of my depressive states went on for months and months and months and I soon became suicidal and began to comfort myself with plans to

THE HUDDLE

kill us and end my awful suffering. I would curl up in a chair, staring at nothing, second after second, minute after minute, day after day, week after week ……. Planning the most effective and foolproof way to bring about my death. I spent hours writing suicide notes and hid them away for Frank to find when I was gone. The thought of being dead was the only thing that comforted me through those dreary days.

It was, however, an evil comfort. It was obviously not doing me any good because I was getting worse and worse and worse. I began to refer to these suicidal plans and arrangements as an 'it' – as a comforter – but an evil one. My evil comforter. 'It' then became a 'he', and I took him unto me like a demon, and he fed on me and drained me. He was killing me and that was exactly what I wanted him to do.

I'd curl up on the floor with him and be convinced that I was already dead and my body was rotting away. I would experience The Huddle as demonic flies, landing on my decaying carcass, feeding off me, picking at my rotten flesh. I still have periods when I 'rot'. Back then I'd take comfort in the certainty that I would soon be really dead as it was not possible to 'exist' this way. The Huddle did, and still do, want me dead, always telling me to kill myself.

"Do everyone a favour you dull bitch and f**king kill your stupid fat fussy frigging self……. She gonna do it one day the fat cow….see how she……."

Dr. Kapp was aware of this evil comforter and told me, implored me, to get rid of him. That is, I had to make a decision to live, however difficult and painful that might be, as Dr. Kapp feared she could not help me unless I gave up the certainty that I would end my life one day soon. I *had* to get rid of him! I cried bitterly. I struggled and fought and hated Dr. Kapp for wanting to take away my only comfort – the knowledge that I could end my miserable existence. I shouted and yelled at her. At one point I ran up the stairs and locked myself in my bedroom, flinging myself, sobbing, onto the bed and refusing to look at her or speak to her. I didn't *want* her telling me to live! To lose my evil comforter would mean choosing to stay alive and live with The Huddle, the terrible depressions, the rotting, Rachel, the others....... As well as seeing to the kids, running a house and going to work!! It was too much! What was I? Bloody Superwoman?? I didn't think so. It was too much to expect of me. I did not want any more of anything. I wanted to be dead.

Eventually, when my mood had lifted a little, Dr. Kapp took me off for the day. It was quite something to feel pampered, looked after and special for a whole day; realising that somebody thought I was worth spending time with in this way.

Then, in a lonely spot high up in the Brecon Beacons Dr. Kapp and I sat and prayed together and I was able to leave my evil comforter up there on the mountain. Out in an open place where he could harm no-one else. I was brought home after a profoundly useful day having made my decision to live, *whatever my life might be like.* There was, much to my surprise, a great deal of relief about this initially, but there have also been many, many

THE HUDDLE

times when I have desperately wanted him back and have cried buckets for the lost comfort of suicidal plans. But suicide must not and can not be. I am a mother. I must point out also that since that day my periods of depression have become much shorter and less severe. How I wished I could have left The Huddle up on top of the Brecon Beacons as well. I certainly tried to – but it was not to be. Why not? I don't know. There is so much that I do not know or understand.

Nowadays when get depressed I cling to nothing, because then there is nothing. Not even an evil comforter. But that's the way it has to be. It is very hard and I can become extremely self pitying. Oh poor me! Why am I like this? I am forever apologising to Frank and my psychiatrist for the way that I am. I am sorry.

Rachel and I once wrote a poem together during a period of depression. What? I'm going to quote yet another chunk of verse? How boring! Well no, not for me, because I'm finding it very therapeutic to sit here typing away. It is helping me not to listen to The Huddle who are, as usual when I sit at my desk, gathered in the desk lamp. This is the poem that we wrote –

Nervous breakdown?
Not for me and not for us!
Not a break *down* but a break *up*!
Into pieces.
I slowly broke up into little pieces.
Slowly.
Painfully.
A slow machete sliced right through my innocence.

Janet Cooper

And now I am me.
Us.
And then this mind depresses itself –
Lower, lower, lower,
Down, down, down,
Until no light be seen.
Darkness and dead agony.
Writhing pain and rot,
And slow decay.
My mind became a dungeon,
Divided into many cells.
In each of which resides
A sad and lonely she.

Horror story people
In the dungeon of my mind,
Clinging to a past
That we can never leave behind.
Too lonely! All the tears
That we can never fully shed
Add thickness to the walls
That keep us separate in this head.

We hate to live together
Yet we cannot live apart,
Both known and unknown side by side,
Frightened, lonely, separate we reside
Together.
But not together.
I'm a paradox.
I'm us.

THE HUDDLE

But now there is an angel in the dungeon of our mind,
Who speaks sweet words of comfort
That ourselves could never find.
She nurtures and encourages
With gentleness, with love.
Enfolds us safe with soft, white wings,
Peace giving,
Like a dove.

Good voice among so many
That are vitriolic, loud.
She a welcome comfort.
They an evil crowd.
Oh! That I and we were able
To leave the bad behind!
Clinging only to an angel
Who's a light within my mind.

You still reading? Want to know what The Huddle are up to now? They are saying that I must rip this typing to shreds.

"She'll rip the s*dding stuff and her piss it into the f**king bin … go shove … she'll … you go ram that b*****d angel up your fat f**king c**t and the devil himself splay you out … he splay her out in his big cathedral and Christ s**t on her, f**k Christ, f**k Christ! What's she doing? She typing wiping s**t on paper and what she say to paper, fat gorgeous little bitch, her witch, you f**king witch … she's sitting s**tting, what she typing? We're here, can't f**king get away, dull bitch……." Etc., etc., etc……….

Charming, eh? I'm not going to apologise for printing this stuff, nor beg you to excuse the language, because if I want this to be an account of The Huddle then it has to be as accurate as my courage allows. It will not help me therapeutically to be euphemistic and tone down what they say. It will not make pleasant reading; it is even less pleasant to live with. At the moment of typing this, I am what I call pretty 'tuned out' of them. That is, I can hear them, I know what they are saying, but I am not listening. Does that make sense? How do I explain? Well, maybe it's like having the radio on while you're busy doing other things. You can hear talking on the radio, and yet you are not actively listening or 'tuned into' the conversation. You can hear it. You know about it. Yet you are apart from it.

I need to have a break from typing now. I am tired and fed up of 'them' in the lamp, snarling away, hating me and staring at me. There is ironing to be done. A change is as good as a rest. Sometimes. It's not too bad when I'm ironing as I keep my brain occupied by listening to music and concentrating on that while they tell me to,

"...hot iron on her fat frigging face and rip the flesh with hell's heat and sweet Christ won't save you .... Burn your p*ssing self, you useless cow ......"

Amazingly, I have never burned myself with an iron! So sorry if you're offended by the language. So am I! You can always stop reading if it gets too bad for you. I can't stop hearing it though!

"What a fanny f**king shame!" They say.

THE HUDDLE

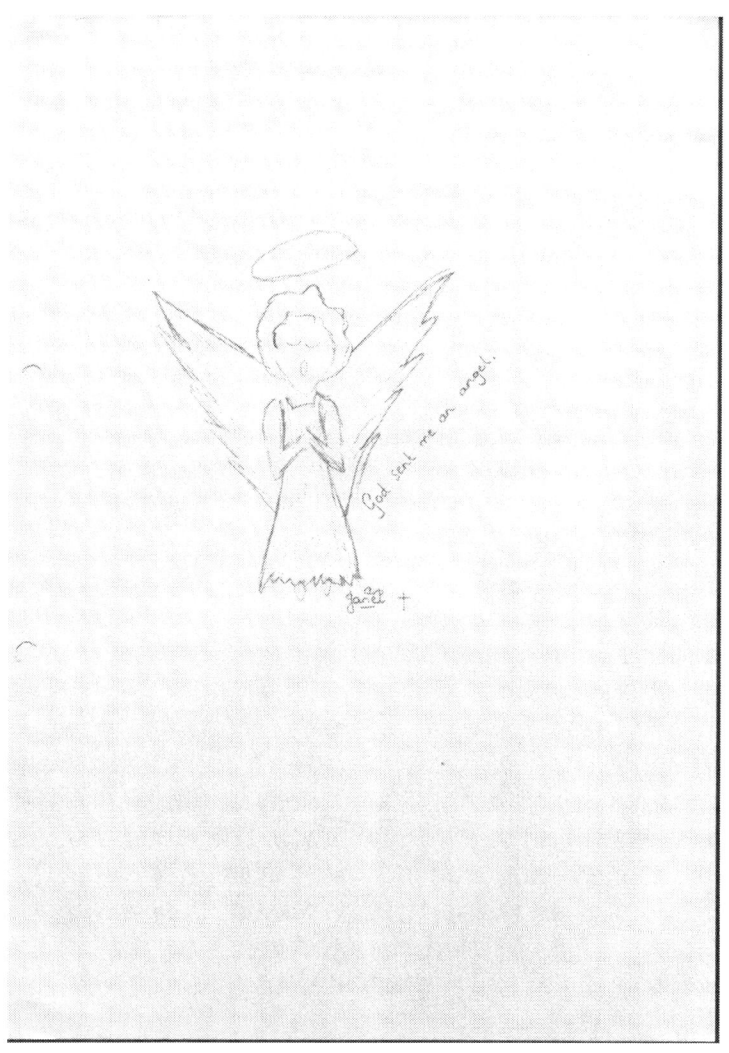

CHAPTER THREE   DEMONS?

When she was with me earlier this week, Dr. Kapp asked me the question she asks during nearly every one of our sessions together.

"What do you think they (The Huddle) are?" I wonder is she expecting me to change my mind at some point? I have, so far, always given the same reply, instantly, often while she is still asking the question.

"DEMONS!!"

During our last session Dr. Kapp also asked me, "Are you hearing them now?" I looked over to the corner of my living-room while I replied in the affirmative, and The Huddle snarled, "Of course she's f**king hearing us! She's always f**king hearing us the poor s*dding cow..." I was able to quickly bring my attention and concentration back to my psychiatrist. But why did I look to the corner of the room? Because that's where they were! Attached to a lamp shade I have a pretty ornamental butterfly, it's actually a fridge magnet, and when I sit in my usual chair The Huddle sound as if they are coming from this little butterfly. Therefore, as far as I'm concerned, they are in the butterfly. I have tried to outwit them by putting the butterfly away in a cupboard but quickly realised that this was a stupid thing to do. It doesn't work. It made them laugh at me while they simply gathered into another object or space.

So they are demons. Right. Why do I say that? Lots of reasons I suppose. So far in this account

THE HUDDLE

I've not quoted them in great detail, but what little I have quoted shows that The Huddle is blasphemous to the extreme. Therefore they are against God, and hate Him. As they are not either flora or fauna then they must belong to some realm of the supernatural. The world of spirits! The Bible describes such anti-Christ entities as devils or demons. Those involved in occult practices would probably refer to them as spirits. Sounds nicer. Good spirits, evil spirits. Angels and demons. So why shouldn't The Huddle be described as demons, or spirits? Radio waves cannot be seen, but they can be heard when received by a receiver, that is, a radio. Demons, spirits, cannot (always) be seen either, but they can be heard by a receiver, by somebody like me. Make any sense? But then I have to ask myself why I am a 'receiver' of these demonic voices? I'm not sure I can give much of an answer to that question, but I'll have a jolly good try!

I have in the past dabbled, or rather plunged into the world of the occult where, driven by fascination and curiosity, I deliberately sought to call up the spirit world, not realising the 'evil' I was also invoking. Too late, I found out that playing these sort of mind games can never be a game. Does this sort of stuff open up channels in the mind, making one prey to this type of phenomena?

I have read two accounts of witches who have wonderfully converted to Christianity and both of those women heard voices. These voices were, for them, successfully dealt with by exorcism. Exorcism did not work for me (Reverend H. blamed me for his inability to deliver me from my demons. I blamed him!!) and maybe an explanation of an involvement in occult activity is not the full answer because it's possible I was already hearing voices before then. However, the occult stuff has not helped my condition in any way and I feel at all times that, because of The Huddle, I am still under the influence of Satan. I am his little puppet and he delights in tormenting me.

I now follow the teachings of Jesus. I love Him! I desire and pine to be able to pray to Him, but it's like a constant battle going on inside my head. The Huddle fights against my mustard seed faith. Satan fights against God, and even though he can never win, the battle is long and vicious. So, although no doubt contributory, my occultism is not the full answer to why I should be receptive to hearing bad voices/demons.

Before I continue with this answer, let me give you an example of the battle that goes on within me. Towards the end of any one day I can be struggling to stay 'tuned out' of The Huddle and just about managing to keep them in the background. Sometimes it can become too much and I become very restless and agitated. It would be impossible to sit and relax and maybe read a book and so I might decide to throw myself into some very energetic housework, to keep myself mentally and physically busy. So,

"What she do now? ... The fat, lazy f**king bitch is CLEANING!! When's sweet Christ gonna clean HER up! Filthy fat freak ...... she stinks! .... You dirty f**king C**t! .... Go piss on the vacuum cleaner, f**k the end of it and f**k Christ ...... God

THE HUDDLE

screw your filthy s**tting fanny ….. Holy f**king cow ….."

I could go on. On and on and on and on and on and ……. Like they do. Are you offended? Me too!

By then, still maybe busy with the frantic housework, I either feel that I shall scream my head off and bang my skull against the nearest concrete wall, or else I have to quickly switch to another coping mechanism before I go completely barmy and the men in white coats come to drag me off. (Becoming psychotic is one of my great fears.) So I might drop the housework and go and sit at the piano instead. What would I play? Most probably a hymn, one of my favourites, 'O Worship the Lord in the Beauty of Holiness'. Beautiful words and lovely music. But you see, the two just don't go together, do they, and I am in agony. It is impossible to worship the Lord in the beauty of holiness when I am in the midst of such blasphemous filth all the time! Agony! I am neither holy nor in the midst of beauty. However, that side of it apart, playing and singing hymns can be very good at calming me down because while my brain is concentrating on several things at one time – reading the music, moving my fingers, singing the words – then I can tune back out of The Huddle,

"F**king glory of merry hell! Not that holy crap again…."

…and they recede once more into the background. Some measure of relief.

But it doesn't work every time. Sometimes, though thankfully not very often, it will make them worse.

"…hypocritical, backslidden, stinking witch! STOP THAT F**KING HOLY ROW!!! …… She go tear up that book NOW. And squeeze the holy words up her p*ssing fanny. … Fat, ugly cow…FAT….UGLY…..COCK SUCKING COW!!!!…………"

Actually I'm not fat, I don't suck male genitals and I'm not a cow. I haven't heard myself moo-ing lately! Ugly? Well, they can be right about some things!

I will never forget the look of terror on my daughter's face one day when The Huddle became worse while I was playing the piano. I suddenly exploded with the frustration of it all. I banged my hands down hard on the piano keys, started screaming hysterically, and began hurling my music books all over the place. Frank rushed in and held me in a bear hug until I was able to get a grip on myself. I was as usual devastated that my daughter had seen me like this yet again. It must be awful to have a mother like me and I worry constantly about the effect I have on my kids. I wish, for their sakes as well as my own sake, that I was not as I am. I love them passionately and tell them so every day. There are masses of cuddles and kisses, and loads of attention when I am able to give it. I am always here for them, as far as I am able to be. But is my overwhelming, unconditional love enough to make it up to them for having me as their mother? My daughter frequently says that she wishes the voices could happen to someone who hasn't got kids –

THE HUDDLE

that cracks me up! I feel so sad and helpless and guilty, and if I could get rid of The Huddle, then I would. Dr. Kapp tells me that I only need to be a 'good enough' mother. I smile sweetly and remain silent while I scream inside my head, 'But I'm NOT a good enough mother! The way I am is not good enough for them!!'

Right. Now to continue an answer to the question I posed earlier on in this chapter. Why should *I* hear voices, spirits demons, whatever you want to refer to them as? (But they are really demons, you know!) Maybe it's because certain events, traumatic to me, damaged my mind at an early age and I came to develop the way I am as some sort of coping mechanism. I had a head full of 'them' rather than having a head full of stuff I didn't want to think about or remember. Remember my five little friends when I was little? The ones who only ever said nice things? Maybe my mind called them into being in order to counteract negative and non nice stuff that was said to me. I remember very clearly a song which used to be sung to me when I was very small. I would be bounced up and down on an Uncle's knee, begging him to sing the 'Janet Bishop is no good' song. How pathetic that I thought that was good and funny! Even more pathetic is that my parents/sister/uncle must also have thought is was funny and okay to sing such words to a little one.

It had a catchy little tune I later was to learn to play on the piano, thus reinforcing the cruel words.

Janet Cooper

"Janet Bishop is no good,
Chop her up for fire wood.
If she is no good for that,
Give her to the pussy cat!"

How appropriate that I should want, instead, nice voices to say nice things to me! So obviously *good* voices can be seen as a defence to the psyche, but surely not the *bad* voices! Or do good voices mutate into bad voices? If so, why and how??? Again, this is not the whole answer to the question.

Let's try another answer. Perhaps I am psychic, possessing the potential to be spiritually aware of a supernatural world, and unfortunately I'm more tuned in to the bad bits! If I am psychic, then presumably I'd be wide open to this type of disturbance. But why me and not somebody else? Same 'luck' as some people being, for example, diabetic, and others not. Same as some people are good at sewing or carpentry or driving a car or singing or making cakes ----- and some people aren't or can't! Personally none of this applies to me except for driving a car. I passed my driving test six years ago after Reverend H. told me I was not safe to walk down the road!! Ya boo to him!! And hang on ….. I do make rather good 'mummy special' chocolate cake which my son tells me is better than Asda's! Praise indeed!

Maybe I'm receptive to the receiving of demonic voices simply because I am. Just because. It might be kinder for me to accept that this is the way I am, rather than torment myself by trying to find the

THE HUDDLE

answer as to why I have The Huddle. I have them because I have them. That's all. Because.

To think of The Huddle as demons, as outside entities, implies that they do not originate within my mind. Same as you can have a cold, but the germs come from outside. It is comforting to think that The Huddle are not *of* me; they are not *Jan* made. If I thought my brain, however involuntarily or subconsciously, was capable of producing this non-stop stream of blasphemies and filth, then I would be hurrying straight back to the Brecon Beacons in search of my evil comforter! Then I would kill myself. I don't think I could live with the knowledge that such obscenity was a part of myself which manifested as voices. By understanding them as outside entities I can at least indulge in a little self pity, oh poor me, rather than succumbing to the fatal misery of knowing I was the author of The Huddle. So as self defence (?) I describe The Huddle as demonic. Therefore they are demons!

During my long exorcism at the hands of Reverend H. it was drummed into me week after week, month after month, that the voices were demons that possessed me. In fact Rev. and Mrs. H. suggested to me, and possibly believed, that everyone who heard voices was possessed.

By demons of course.

Psychiatric hospitals apparently contain schizophrenics with heads full of devils! No doubt it feels that way for these tortured souls. I wouldn't know. I am neither schizophrenic (a common assumption about voice hearers) nor am I possessed. I wonder what Rev. and Mrs. H. would have made of Angel? If it is possible to be possessed by demons, then wouldn't it be possible to be possessed by angels? Ha! I am positive that they would describe her as an angel of darkness come clothed as an angel of light! They would still insist I was demon possessed.

I would like to drop the word 'possession', whilst still allowing that everything I have been taught about the character of demons is indeed applicable to The Huddle.   i.e. They hate God, they hate me, they are exceptionally blasphemous, they seek to spoil and destroy my life, they are in total opposition to Christianity and they are profoundly evil towards anything that God has made, especially humans who are made in his image. God made me.

The Huddle react violently when I read my Bible, I find it almost impossible to pray, they have driven me to cut myself, starve myself to the point of severe anorexia, and try to kill myself. There is no good in them whatsoever. Only evil. They are demonic in character. They are demons! Sounds like a reasonable, sensible and accurate description. Well it does to me, anyway. What does Dr. Kapp think the voices are? She doesn't say. Probably because she doesn't know herself, and it's hard for Dr.s to admit they don't know something!

Dr. Kapp used to get me to think of the voices as loops of tape inside my head going on and on and on and on. This helped temporarily. But they are not always inside my head! They huddle in objects, in ornaments; they occupy spaces and follow me by occupying the space around or behind my head. I hear them with my ears, same as

THE HUDDLE

another person speaking to me. That person is not literally inside my head, even though that's where my ears will take their voice. Neither is The Huddle literally inside my head. Am I making any sense, I wonder? I know what I mean but find it difficult to put down on paper. Thick as a plank creature that I am!

The Huddle are now agreeing loudly with that last sentence, and so time for a break from the typewriter.

"…and break it over your f**king lousy head and go and make your stupid coffee you stupid slurping f**king cow you! ….. We'll f**king get you girlie! … Fat frigger ……"

Well no. I'm neither fat nor masturbatory. But I am gasping for a cuppa!!

Coffee break over. I haven't just had a cup of coffee however. I needed to tune back out of The Huddle in order to carry on with this account, and so put on a video of an aerobic workout and leapt energetically around my living-room. This also helps when I'm angry, as focusing on the movements, the music, and the television occupies my brain. A few endorphins rushing about and The Huddle are well and truly in the background. I have the added advantage with this coping mechanism that it is also good for my cardiovascular system and keeps my weight stable. Not bad eh? Now what was I on about? Had I been writing about Rev.H?

Janet Cooper

Now I was told by the Reverend that if I was ever to consult a psychiatrist ("A psychiatrist can't help you Janet!"), then I would most probably be diagnosed as having Multiple Personality Disorder. "It's another name for demon possession Janet! You need to be delivered, and I can help you." (Arrogant twit!) That is, he was going to carry out major exorcisms again and again and again. He was to keep going despite the fact that I was getting worse and worse and worse. But exorcism was most certainly not the answer. It was abusive to say the least and psychiatry has treated me in a more Godly way. Dr. Kapp has respected the human being that I am in the midst of all this turmoil. She has never ever abused me or made me worse, the way exorcism did. Psychotherapy has supported and nurtured me and I am better able to cope than I have ever been. It is a long journey, but one of hope and healing.

Exorcism only plunged me to the depths of a hell I am still struggling out of. Am I being unkind to the Reverend who tried to help me? I don't think so. Remember that I was severely depressed, profoundly suicidal, hearing voices and severely anorexic and underweight. Would you say that a minister of a Baptist chapel was trained to cope, alone, with someone like this? He never even told me to see my G.P.!! He surely should have realised that I needed expert help, yet blindly, proudly(?) carried on with his wretched 'treatment'. At the time I was in too much of a state to question him. It was as if Frank and I were under some sort of spell, captured by this man's authoritative personality, and were compelled to go along with him. We were

THE HUDDLE

vulnerable. I was ill. My stepfather 'threatened' to phone Reverend H. and sort him out, but never did. It was an awkward and confusing time. I think I'm waffling again, but so what. It doesn't matter. This is *my* book. I can write what I like.

Another question I would like to ask you, dear reader, is this. If The Huddle are *not* demons, then what are they? I have at times been able to see them, so therefore they have to exist outside of myself, and they don't look good. They look evil. They look exactly how I would expect demons to look. Aha! You've quickly latched on to that one! They are an hallucination that originates in my mind because I have an idea of what I expect a demon to look like. Therefore that's what I see when I see them. Visual hallucinations! But don't forget that if I see something that you cannot see, then that something is real to me, so as far as I am concerned it exists. You cannot prove to me it doesn't, any more than I can prove to you it does! It is unverifiable! Like God! So is there something peculiar or 'wrong' with me because I can see it, or is there something peculiar about *you*? Are you defective in some way because you *can't* see it?

I've never thought of myself as having hallucinatory tendencies because what I see and hear is very real to me. It is *my* reality. Is The Huddle a group of auditory hallucinations? No. Because they are real to me, they exist; they have an effect in my life. It actually never ceases to amaze me that Dr. Kapp has never heard The Huddle, after all the time she has spent with me and them. They are right there, next to where she sits on my settee. What is wrong with her that she cannot hear them? Frank has, at times, been able to sense what they are saying to me, particularly when I am disturbed and upset by them. Why, why, why can't other people hear them when they are so real??

I suppose all this leads to that major philosophical puzzle – what is reality? From my side of the fence, who is more in touch with the real reality of existence? The voice hearers or you other lot out there? What, oh what, is reality??? A whopping big subject, that's for sure, and one I'm not clever enough to have a stab at in any depth. But I do know that The Huddle are real – argue with me by all means – but they are *my* reality! They are demons. They look and act and speak and hate. Just like demons.

Another reason why I say they are demons is because The Huddle themselves say that they are!

"F**king right we do, foul demons vomited from merry hell, her belly swell with s**t from hell we tell sweet Christ to f**ky off and Satan shoves his c**k right up her p*ssing little......."

They refer to Satan as their master and my master, and as being more powerful than God who I attempt to pray to. They describe themselves as God's enemies and hate Him venomously. They are my enemies also, and absolutely, utterly detest me. 'Consider mine enemies for they are many and hate me with cruel hatred.' (Psalm 25:19) The Huddle know that they are evil.

"F**king quite correct we know it! Stupid s*dding c**t! Father f**king freak!"

Doesn't that sound demonic to you?

THE HUDDLE

"F**k sweet Christ and s**t on His b***ard cross you dull c**t, with runt, suck his frigging c**k and go vomit on His p*ssing ugly face, she go and bleed all over……."

Well doesn't it? If those words are not evil, then what the hell words are?? I would point out here that nowhere in this account will I quote the very worst of what they say. Why not? Because I am ashamed to be hearing it, and of my ability to hear it. It frightens me. It is polluting and unedifying. It should not be written down in black and white, it is so hateful and destructive. But people who don't hear voices but want to understand why it causes such distress *need* to see some of the crap these things spew out night and day. It's okay to say they swear, they're not nice – but what *do* they say??? I hope, sadly, that you now have some idea, albeit gleaned only from *my* experience.

I took the following from Psalms 69 and 70.

"They that hate me without a cause are more than the hairs on my head. They that would destroy me, being mine enemies wrongfully, are mighty … I am in trouble, draw nigh unto my soul, deliver me because of mine enemies. I am full of heaviness. ('you're also full of F**king s**t, she holy s*dding cow and…..') Let them be ashamed and confounded who seek after my soul, let them be turned backward and put to confusion who desire my hurt. I am poor and needy. O God, be Thou my help and deliverer."

Please!! I could pray so many of the Psalms against The Huddle, taking them to be the enemy about which the psalmist writes.

Janet Cooper

"Holy God quoting bitch! She fill that f**king head with Christ sweet crap and go and s**t sweet music to the King, you fat, ugly cow, go f**k off!..." Etc. I have never heard a human being speak this way. Maybe some people do! But are they capable of keeping it up twenty four hours a day?

It is again becoming difficult to type. They are too noticeable to me again and so I must take another break. My concentration is not good now. Go do something else. I cannot rest. I must employ one of my coping mechanisms until they recede once more into the background.

I want to curl up on a chair
And die.
But cry
Because I can't.
I mustn't.
So I won't.
Somebody help me, please?

Deep, deep pools of terrible despair,
Down and down and down.
But not to death,
To nothing.
Absolutely nothing.
I am nothing.
But they are them.
And there are others,
Plus an angel
In the dungeon of my mind.

"Poor little f**king cow you are, she is, s*dding hate you! Fat freak! Stop typing, stop typing,

THE HUDDLE

stoptypingstoptypingstop………." And if I didn't stop typing any time soon then they would be capable of chanting that at me for hours. I can now also hear Rachel. She is lying on the floor of her cell and crying bitterly. She wishes she was dead. Janny wants to see the mouse. "Can I play? I go and play mouse. Give them a smooth."

Dear head,
         Why are you so dark and noisy and busy now? Why can't I ever have a rest? Why don't The Huddle and you all go away? Please leave me alone for I can't take much more. Yet what choice do I have?

"How long O Lord wilt Thou look on?" Jesus says "Come!" but I run a mile because of The Huddle and because there are too many of me and because I am unacceptable to God in the state that I am in. Why doesn't God make us better?

Head? I hate you! Go away!!
    From Janet.

I am so very sorry for the way that I am. Must stop typing now. Getting too hard and sooooooo slow. Too slow.

If I was deaf, would I still hear The Huddle???????????????

Janet Cooper

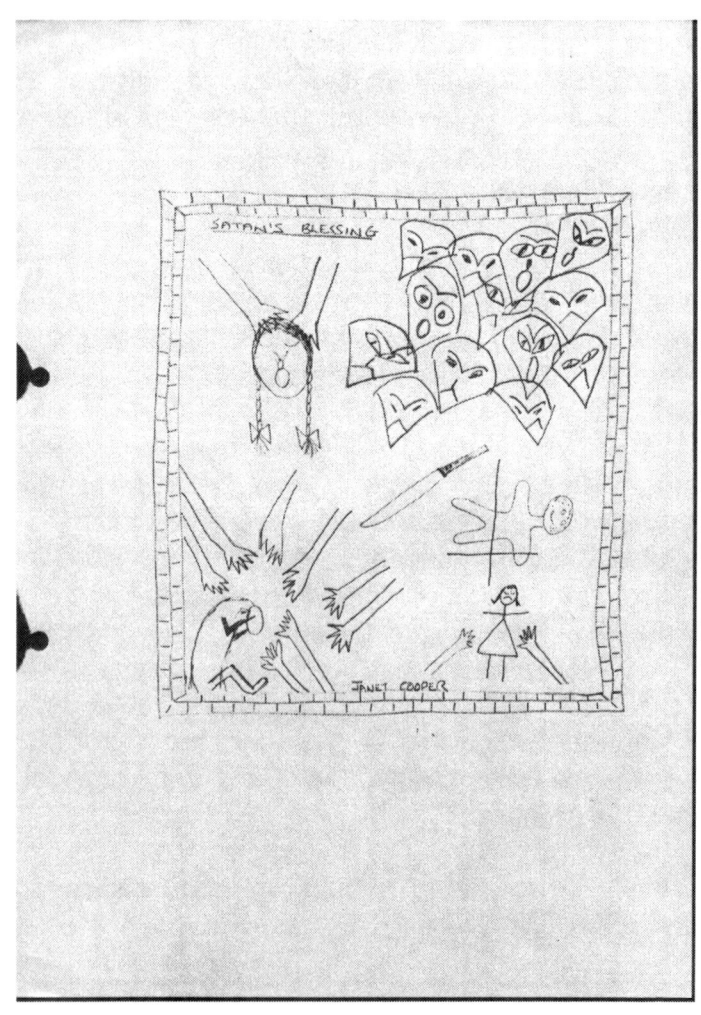

THE HUDDLE

CHAPTER FOUR   A LONELY AND SECRET MALADY

Malady: any disease or illness. Haven't I written previously that I do not think of myself as being ill? Yes. And I'm going to stick to that even though at times I do feel ill with it all. Think positive eh? But you must agree that I most certainly do experience a degree of dis-ease. According to the Collins dictionary which lies open beside me, the word 'malady' also means any unhealthy, morbid or desperate condition. Oh? So maybe I am ill with it! Now I've got myself thoroughly confused and wishing I'd chosen a different title for this chapter. ("So go f**king change it, dull cow!") But no problem! All I wanted to say was that my condition (malady?) is a lonely one that I feel is wise to be secretive about.

I do not *look* as if I hear voices. What does a voice hearer look like for goodness sake? Vague? Haunted? Not quite human? Different? A knife wielding, people slashing lunatic? Some comments I've received go like this;
Anybody in there?   (Yeh! A few of us!!)
You're in a world of your own.   (True!)
Are you with us?
Have you heard a word I've said?
Are you alright?
Snap out of it!
She's off again.
Come back to us!

Few people know why I act in such a way so as to invite these sorts of comments. That is because I keep the fact that I hear voices a secret. Why?

Janet Cooper

Many people associate hearing voices with Schizophrenia and will immediately remember a news article where some poor tormented soul has, under the direction of voices, lashed out, hurting or even killing somebody. Please know that the vast majority of violent crimes are committed by people who *don't* hear voices – yet there is no stigma attached to non voice hearers!! That seems a bit unfair to me. Hearing voices is something most people know nothing about; it is alien to them and they do not understand. Voice hearers are not crazy killing machines ready to spring into action when the going gets tough! My violent outbursts have only ever been against myself, and although I am told several times a day to kill Frank, he's not afraid to sleep in the same bed! There is still so much stigma attached to mental illness and hearing voices would seem go hand in hand with being mentally ill. This is not necessarily so! Nor is hearing voices something that is easy to talk about. It doesn't exactly crop up in everyday conversations. For example, how about this? –

"Hello! How are you?" Common enough salutation.
"Fine thanks, apart from this lousy cold I've got, fed up of coughing all the time!" Common enough answer in bug infested Britain. And that's okay! Get a bit of sympathy and understanding for your lousy cold. Most people know about colds. Another example –

"Hello! How are you?"
"I'm doing okay thanks, but these lousy voices are really getting me down." What would the reaction

THE HUDDLE

be? Would I get the same sympathy and understanding? Or would I be on the receiving end of a blank look and a polite smile followed by an embarrassed, don't know what to say, silence?

Can you imagine the children telling their friends in school that their mother hears voices?

"So and so's mother hears voices! She must be nuts!"

It's hardly the same as saying your mum has diabetes, or a headache, or a broken big toe! It is wiser to keep it secret.

Only a very few of the people I'm in contact with now know about The Huddle. Frank and the children know, my mother knows, and two neighbours we are particularly friendly with know. They know because my son has had to run to them in emergencies, when I am cut, covered in blood, and not 'with it' enough to see to myself. Obviously my psychiatrist knows.

Frank and I have no social life whatsoever as it saves having to explain my sometimes odd behaviour which can make me appear ignorant, rude, and stand offish. I do not have any close friends. Couldn't cope! Would such a relationship necessitate at least a brief explanation of my condition? How else would I explain my refusal to answer the telephone, my sudden depressions, my frequent inability to answer my own front door, and my elective muteness which can last anything from several hours to (on one occasion) several months? The Huddle has turned me into a very lonely and solitary person.

I wrote this in my diary not so very long ago. –

"We are all tired and I don't know what will happen to me. Truth? I want to be dead for I cannot see any other way out of my mind. I don't know how long I can go on appearing to be alright. It is wearing me out and I never feel alright and they are making me so tired and I am frightened and I am lonely and nobody understands. I am too lonely. Hosts encamp around me. I am sad. It is time to go to bed. The Huddle will follow me. It is so very, very lonely."

Another neighbour, who lives opposite to us, came over for a chat one warm, sunny day.
"Haven't done much to the garden this year, have you?" He didn't mean it critically, but as a keen gardener, anyone who 'only' mows the lawn and keeps things generally tidy isn't really gardening. However, my hackles rose and I could cheerfully have bopped him one! But what he said was true! I had been too busy trying to struggle through each day and cope with The Huddle in the hope of not going nuts and ending up in hospital again. Maybe he would not have made such a comment if my malady had been a visible one, such as a broken leg encased in a sympathy inducing cast!

Secret and lonely. So lonely……..

Last August Frank and I took the kids to Bristol Zoo. I happen to hate the place, believing it to be cruel to cage animals, but the kids loved it and enjoyed their visit, which made it so worth the effort! When we reached the elephant compound I

THE HUDDLE

was reduced to hiding my tears by the sight of a huge elephant called Wendy, standing all alone, sad looking, while people gathered around, staring at her and talking about her. I felt an instant connection with her, sharing her loneliness, and when I was back at home that evening I wrote this,

Dear Wendy,
        The Huddle had followed me all the way up the M4 and I found myself looking at you and knowing maybe a little more than most about how you might be feeling. Sad and alone and lost. There was only one of you. None other like you in the whole zoo. I feel like there is only one of me because I've never met anyone else who hears voices and has others inside their head.

Your compound was pleasant enough and safe for you, if on the small side. Like my home. That is safe for me. Your compound was also completely escape proof. My head is like that. I cannot escape. I cannot truly escape my home either because I'm not 'allowed' in other people's houses, same as you're not allowed into other animals compounds. Neither of us is free in any way.

I looked at your eyes and they were so sad. Very small, too. Almost too small for your great size, as if you needed not to see too much of the world. Like my Katy. Rachel says that Katy does not want or need to see the world. Are you like that?

My eyes filled with tears and I ached for you in your loneliness. Damn that zoo! Yet you were surrounded; constantly surrounded by spectators. By faces. Everywhere. Looking at you. I have faces looking at me too. You were also surrounded by voices. Lots of huddles! Huddles of people talking about you, to you, calling out, shouting, laughing…….. It's horrid, isn't it! Kids laughing and sniggering and being vulgar because you have to excrete in front of them. There is never any privacy, is there? My voices are cruel like that. They watch and talk and laugh and make comments when I go to the loo. Even if I lock the door it's still like performing in front of an audience! You and me. We are lonely and yet never alone.

I watched as you ate some hay. Why the hell do you eat? Is it because, like me, you have some deeply subconscious drive to keep your body alive? And your voices yelled at you,

"Look! She's eating! Wow! Look how much she's putting in her mouth! Isn't she a greedy guts!"

Just like The Huddle. Except they swear a lot too.

Maybe you don't know about the possibility of being dead, what a release it would be from your cruel, unnatural situation. I long for this release, but there are people who want me and need me to stay alive. Like people want you to stay alive – to serve a purpose for them. For their need and pleasure. Not yours or mine.

At noon you were taken for a brief stroll around the grounds, but still you were a captive. As you did as you were told and allowed, your 'voices' followed you. Incessantly followed! Nowhere on earth to be quiet and alone.

I have a psychiatrist. I suppose you have a vet who visits you regularly to keep you okay, the way Dr. Kapp seeks to keep me okay. Does your vet

THE HUDDLE

make you feel cared for? My psychiatrist does. You will have a vet for the rest of your life but Dr. Kapp won't be with me for much longer and then …….. Do you like your vet? I like Dr. Kapp but sometimes I want to hate her because if it was not for her then I would be dead. I should be grateful, and sometimes I am. Then sometimes I'm not. Do you have feelings like that? Do you long for a friend, a real friend? Is your vet a real friend because he knows so much about you? Hey, that's only because he's read the books and learned how to handle you! Is he really a friend...

If you were released you would not know how to survive. It would be kinder to destroy you. Captives or free, our lot is to live in a hell. One day I shall be mad. I plan to be dead before that happens.

Wendy is a funny name for an elephant. It conjures up an image in my mind of somebody small and cute and pretty. Maybe we can both be that in our dreams.

What do you dream about? Do you manage to escape the voices at night when it is cool and dark? Or does the memory of it all return to haunt you again and again and again? Are you, even in slumber, incessantly followed? So you wake up to escape the dream, only to realise that there *is* no escape. Ever! Only another day to get through. Somehow.

Wendy? Do you forgive those who keep you in this state? Do you forgive the faces and the voices for their rude and personal remarks? For their shouting and laughing and sniggering? Do you hate your life and yet know no different?

Janet Cooper

I feel so sorry for you and wish with all my heart that you had never been born for this existence. Tonight, in a dream, we shall wander out into the wilderness together. You and me. Two lonely creatures. We shall look for the only true friend. We will look for Jesus.
Then, and only ever then… Amen.
    With love,
      Janet.

When I had finished this letter, Rachel wanted to write one too. "Me write too!" This is her letter.

Dear Tiger,
    You are so very beautiful and I am so f**king ugly. I saw you, I did, pacing back and forth in your cell but there was not any way out, was there. You didn't see anything while you were pacing. Pacing. Pacing. You looked tired of it and also frustrated as if you were having a nervous breakdown and about to go **MAD** like me. I am not allowed out and I feel like I am going **NUTS**!!!!!!!!!! And the voices all talking about us and looking at us and it is not a good way for us to be and
    I WISH WE WERE
        BOTH
           STONE
               <u>DEAD</u>!!!!!!!
        Luv,
           Rachel.

Me again now. Janet. When I go to bed at night the last words I will hear are,

THE HUDDLE

"Bitch is going to sleep now ….. Bitch go sleep ….. Lazy f**king bitch!"

It can be hours before I finally sleep as I lie there trying not to listen to them. Often I will turn to where they are. In my bedroom The Huddle will settle themselves into the gap between the panes of glass in the double glazed window. Frank knows where they are and is sympathetic about my struggle to sleep, understanding why I'm so restless and constantly tossing and turning. Often he will sit and rock me when I break down and cry because I'm so fed up. But I can hardly begin to describe the loneliness that descends upon me when Frank eventually sleeps and I am left awake with The Huddle for company. Rachel will often be awake with me, but she is hardly pleasant company! Never alone, but so painfully lonely.

The house will be dark and still, my family peaceful in slumber, everyone asleep but us and The Huddle. Who is there that will be with me and comfort me?

"I cried unto God with my voice, even unto God with my voice ……in the day of my trouble I sought the Lord: My sore ran in the night, and ceased not, my soul refused to be comforted. I remembered God and was troubled: I complained and my spirit was overwhelmed. Thou holdest mine eyes waking. I am so troubled that I cannot speak." (From Psalm 77) "Keep not Thou silent, O God. Hold not thy peace and be not still, O God. For, lo, Thine enemies make a tumult: and they that hate Thee have lifted up the head." (From Psalm 83)

So many of the Psalms can become prayers for me. Listen to this one. See how appropriate it is to my condition.

"Give ear to my prayer, O God: and hide not thyself from my supplication. Attend unto me, and hear me: I mourn in my complaint and make a noise; because of the voice of the enemy, because of the oppression of the wicked: For they cast iniquity upon me, and in wrath they hate me. My heart is sore pained within me: and the terrors of death are fallen upon me. Fearfulness and trembling are come upon me, and horror hath overwhelmed me. And I said, O that I had wings like a dove! For then I would fly away, and be at rest." (Psalm 56:1-6) I love that last verse. O to have the wings of a dove.......

The only flying I do in the middle of a night is down a flight of stairs! Night after night after night I get up once or twice sometimes for several hours at a time. The children don't know about it. Frank is not aware of the true extent of my wakefulness.

"Get out of that f**king bed you cock sucking slovenly cow! She get up in a minute ... got to get up, lazy bitch, ... get up out of that stinking bed ... get up ... she get up now .... Get up....GET UP BITCH!!!!"

So I get up, because I cannot stand to have to lie there listening to them with nothing to distract me. Also, if Frank is asleep, or almost asleep, I get up to give him a bit of peace. He has to get up for work five mornings a week and it would be grossly unfair of me to keep him awake when I can't settle down anyway.

THE HUDDLE

My overwhelming complaint about these dark and sleepless hours is one of utter loneliness, and I dare say I share this feeling with many of the world's insomniacs. I am aware of the others in my head. I have The Huddle. The cat is usually curled up on a chair. The gerbils will be busy in their tank beneath the television. I am indescribably lonely. God knows. But I find it so hard to share with Him. The Huddle won't let me. As soon as I try to think prayer words, they will over-ride them with their scatological, blasphemous filth.

Often in the middle of the night I will sit and write to Dr. Kapp, just to feel that I'm in touch with somebody who understands how I am probably better than anyone else does. I might tell her that it's 2.37a.m., it's cold, the cat's asleep, The Huddle is driving me nuts, Rachel is still not speaking to me, I've just had a cup of tea …… It must make such boring reading, page after page. Dr. Kapp is so patient with me about all this.

Or else I might employ another of my coping mechanisms and sit cross legged on the floor, headphones on, listening to music. Usually my top favourites – Mozart's Requiem, Vivaldi's Gloria, or anything by J.S.Bach. Beautiful, beautiful music and singing. Music is one of my most successful coping mechanisms, enabling me to tune well out of The Huddle.

But most often, because I'm too tired to cope, too lonely but never alone in the middle of the night, I will curl up on the floor and rot. I will find myself sinking, sinking, ever lower and lower, into despair so great and painful that it is not possible to suffer such torment and remain alive. This sort of agony is in no way compatible with life and so I will become dead and rotting. Endless, thickest blackness and nothingness. No other way to describe this sort of depression. The pain defies description so that I can only bear it by dying. I stink and decay. The smell is awful and The Huddle will be flies and maggots, landing on me, attacking me, picking on me, and crawling over my rotting carcass. I am dead to the world; just as The Huddle want me to be. A decaying, rotting, stinking, offensive carcass that is a contaminant to its surroundings. Utterly useless and unwanted. Lying on the floor and then kicked into a corner. Time stands still and I will never live again……

(Grim stuff, dear reader. Had enough?? Yeh. Me too…….)

I do eventually get back to bed most nights and hopefully manage a few hours much needed sleep. Later on when I awaken, the first words I hear, every single day, without fail, are,
"Bitch is awake!" Some people start the day with a bowl of cornflakes and a slice of toast. I start the day with The Huddle and a torrent of filth.
"Every day they wrest my words: all their thoughts are against me for evil. They gather themselves together, they hide themselves, they mark my steps, when they wait for my soul." (Psalm 56:5, 6) "O God, my God, put thou my tears into thy bottle … when I cry unto thee, then shall mine enemies turn back…" (Psalm 56:8, 9) Oh! That The Huddle would be turned back! I try so hard to pray, to pray to God, but maybe I'm not trying hard

enough, or maybe my tears are too full of self pity. The Huddle render me prayerless and I cannot speak words to Him.

"Mine enemies would daily swallow me up: for they be many that fight against me." (Psalm 56:2) Lonely and secret suffering, night after night, only to wake up to go through more of it, day after day. The psalmist writes,

"Weeping may endure for a night but joy cometh in the morning." (Psalm 30:5) But joy does not come to me in the morning! But yet some measure of relief does, because I am no longer dead and rotting. Not until the next night, anyway. Maybe 'morning' refers to the start of a new life when I shall no longer have The Huddle.

But what do I do NOW? Have hope? Or despair of ever getting rid of them? Go totally barmy? Kill myself? Scream my head off? WHAT THE BLOODY HELL AM I TO DO?????????

"Cast thy burden upon the Lord and he shall sustain thee." (Psalm 55:22)

Will He?? How!!??!!

Allow me now to do a little rambling, off and away from the subject of this chapter but still relevant to this book.

Last Saturday I was keeping very busy and so had managed to stay quite tolerably tuned out of The Huddle. I awoke. (Bitch is awake!) I tried to lie in, (Slovenly cow ... get up or she get screwed ... lazy bitch ... she have to get up ...) but couldn't, so got up and had breakfast (Fat friggin' glutton!). I then spent some time doing the washing, hanging it on the line and tidying around, making breakfast for Frank and the kids, and sorting them out after which we all piled into the car to take my son to Cardiff, as he was to spend the day with a friend who lives on a farm there. It is a constant delight to me that my son and my daughter have so many friends and such a busy social life. That has never applied to their mother! Anyway, from there, three of us ended up in Caerphilly Garden Centre. Santa's Grotto was in full swing and most of the inside was given over to the baubles and trappings of a merry Christmas to one and all.

I was thrilled to see my daughter's face light up as she browsed around and I was able to enjoy her excitement. The Huddle, however, were not thrilled. Predictably *un*thrilled!

"So it's the birthday of sweet f**king Christ, why don't you get the hell out of here? What you doin' here? ...Shouldn't be here, she shouldn't be here, don't deserve, what she gonna do? ... buy sweet Christ a Christmas tree angel to f**k or......"

I continued to walk with Frank and my daughter around the various displays. I was fine. I could hear them but I was fine.

"F**king bells of merry hell! Why don't you ram those pretty witty balls right up your p*ssing little......"

I'd just about had enough of being fine while all this was going on when we arrived at the café. Hubby and I had a coffee each.

"Liquid f**king s**t! ... She drinks the blood from the cup of the devil and the whole of heaven hates

THE HUDDLE

her, you belong to our master in hell … she drinks and winks and stinks….."

My daughter sat quietly sipping orange juice and eating crisps. A normal looking family outing. I was offered a crisp. Crunch! (As crisps do so wonderfully!)

"Hear her s*dding bones crunching, that's what we'll f**king do to you, dull c**t, crush bones, eat the f**king crunched bones, foetus bones, the wild and wicked witch and….."

After that delightful little rest (I *am* being sarcastic!) we had a last look around at the Christmas stuff. They always put on a fantastic display! Everything was so pretty and sparkly.

"F**k the bloody lot of this! We go smash it to bits … smash the f**king lot to merry hell all holy garbage clap trap f**k Christ rubbish s**t fat git … and smash and trash and smash and trash and … happy birthday to him … go f**k him, go f**k him, go f**k him…"

As we made our way back to the car I unfortunately noticed a pile of dog mess on the ground.

"God! Eat it! Slimy turd, get word, eat it! … she's going to eat it…..EAT IT NOW!!!!!"

I closed my eyes and screwed my face up for a few seconds to get the nasty out of my head.

For the whole of that visit The Huddle had not shut up and had remained in the space around my head except for when we were sat in the café when they moved into a nearby wall picture. This, believe it or not, had actually been a rather good outing. At least I had got out of the car. At least I had not felt desperate and driven to cut our visit short. At least I was able to enjoy seeing the pleasure on my daughter's face, and really, this *does* fit into the title of this chapter, because my part of the visit was secret.

Nobody else knew what was going on with regards to the Huddle. I felt lonely to be hearing them, like I was detached from everyone and everything, nursing some awful secret about what the world was really like. What the hell was the matter with everyone else at the garden centre that they weren't hearing The Huddle? Doesn't the Bible tell us concerning the spiritual realm that there are ten thousand on our right and just as many on our left? I can hear a handful of them, so why can't the rest of you? What's wrong with you all??

Maybe somebody else there *was* hearing voices! How would I know? What does a voice hearer look like? Normal? What's normality anyway? Are people who kill themselves more 'normal' than the rest of us in that they refuse to put up with this crazy world we live in?

Nobody is immune from suffering. You, dear reader, might hear voices one day. How do you know that you won't? Because you are strong? Healthy? Have a high IQ? You're a professional? You're well off? You belong to the socio-economic group that is less likely to hear voices? Hogwash! That doesn't exclude you. Joan of Ark heard voices, so did Jesus, so did Spike Milligan, so do other famous people. I'm kicking myself now because I can't remember their names, but there is a long list of them!!

Given a choice, I would choose to have a physical illness instead of The Huddle, the others,

THE HUDDLE

and my horrible depressions and rotting. If I suffered from arthritis, diabetes, cancer (even though it might be fatal – so might The Huddle!), deformed feet, whatever….. Then I would at least be open to a bit of sympathy and understanding. Do I sound snivellingly, self pitying, as if I don't understand the extent of physical suffering? Do you? Do you also understand the extent of mental pain?

Maybe it's easier to suffer when you can share it with more people, being totally open about your malady and having a socially acceptable reason for its effects and limitations. Maybe you are of the opinion that physical pain is much worse than mental pain and cannot possibly be compared to depression or hearing voices. So *is* physical pain worse? Prove it!

In the case of a terminal illness in which great pain is suffered, the sufferer is assured of an end to his wretched state by virtue of the fatality of his condition. However bad the pain, the end is in sight. Minus my evil comforter I do not have an end in sight! I can only see it going on and on and on and on and there are so many days when I cry bitterly and angrily. I wouldn't know how effective analgesia is for chronic pain these days, but medication has unfortunately not been very helpful in my case.

Perhaps my neighbour would not have commented on my lack of gardening if I'd had a physical illness I could explain and be open about. Maybe another Mum would then offer to collect my daughter from school when it's tipping down with rain. (Why should she, I hear you ask. For the same reason I collected her kids one awful day when she was ill with flu!) The Huddle detest rain and make it a misery for me to go out in it. Can you imaging explaining that to the teacher?

"I'm collecting Heather today because her Mum's voices don't like the rain."

Frequently I shed more tears than the sky.

(Right! I'm off on a pity party here, so if you don't want to come then shut the book! That's okay with me. You remain comfortable and undisturbed!)

If I was physically ill and had a really bad couple of weeks there is the possibility of a get well card and a bunch of grapes. Of being able to share. Then when I was having good weeks there would be admiration at my ability to cope and put up with my lot.

"Isn't she wonderful, the way she copes, hardly ever complains."

I am *not* wonderful in the way I cope and I complain bitterly. But only to my psychiatrist. I try not to complain much to Frank because it must be hard to live with a self pitying wretch like me, without me moaning ad infinitum.

If my malady was purely physical then perhaps it would not have denied me the privilege of friends and a social life. Friends to share problems and joys with. For company. To talk nicely! But I don't have a visible and therefore more acceptable malady. I have The Huddle and they are totally unacceptable. The Huddle affect me mentally and so instead of wallowing in the sympathy of others, I wallow in the mud of my own self pity.

THE HUDDLE

"The dog returns to its vomit, Janet." Reverend H quoted that to me from the Bible. Thanks mate……

My only mental help and support comes from my psychiatrist. We sit and we talk and she is so very patient with me. I'm very fond of her and don't know what I'll do without her. But she isn't somebody I could call on to whisk the kids away for an hour or two when I am sat on the floor rocking, crying and holding my head in my hands. I don't have help in this way or in other ways when physical help would have lightened the load somewhat. Nevertheless, the attention of my psychiatrist is an enormous privilege of which I am very aware. She has literally been my lifeline. I have her. Frank has nobody and he has to live with us. Should have typed 'me' there, but I *am* an us.

Not long after we married I had an abdominal operation. I came home and was under the weather for a few weeks. Neighbours called, cards arrived, colleagues phoned, flowers and chocolates arrived, all of which cheered me up and made me feel better.

How different it was when I was rushed into St. Cadoc's! I was also under the weather for many weeks when I came home. This time there was not one card, one flower, one comforting little choccy or one bloody grape! Why not? Well, psychiatric hospital. Stigma! Nervous breakdown? Snap out of it. Why doesn't she pull herself together? What did I have to be depressed about? What indeed. Met The Huddle lately? Or Rachel? Or Katy, or…….

Now that I've said all that, I'm going to rebuke myself. Such complaining can't be helpful to me and yet it has been cathartic to write it down. The thing is, when I am depressed I reject people anyway, what few there are around me to reject! It is difficult to be friends with somebody who periodically refuses to speak, answer the telephone or open the front door. I can be joyless, unsmiling, boring, lazy and indifferent. In other words, I'm a miserable bloody pig! Little wonder I miss out on the sympathy and choccies when I have a bad couple of weeks – I wouldn't want them anyway! And what have I done to deserve such attention? What could I give in return? I would not be capable of being a friend because friendship is a two way thing and I see absolutely nothing whatsoever that I have to offer a potential friend that is worth giving. Dr. Kapp would strongly disagree with that statement but I know I'm right. I am not worth making friends with because when people found out what I was really like then they would not want to know me. Would you? There is nothing of myself worth giving.

Okay. That's the end of *that* particular pity party. Time to close this chapter I think.

"You can close the whole f**king book if you want to! ….. She going to write more? …she write more s**t rubbish…"

Yes. You bet I'm going to write more! Much more. I haven't finished yet. I'm going to write you

THE HUDDLE

out of my head and I'm starting to get very angry…… but just one last moan before I type my neat little line. (This will be the doggy bag after the party!!)

Why is it that if somebody dies from cancer then that is seen as a more acceptable death than if somebody dies of depression (i.e. suicide)? Both are potentially fatal illnesses (could we not even refer to depression as a cancer of the mind?) yet consider the difference in the deaths column of your local newspaper.

Following terminal cancer,
"After much suffering borne with great dignity," "After a long brave fight," "After an illness borne with great courage," Etc.

That's okay, that's fine, and I'm certainly not saying that this is inappropriate and that the deceased did not deserve such commentary – far from it. (And bear in mind that some cancers are self induced! I'm thinking particularly about the lifelong heavy smoker who ignored all the 'SMOKING KILLS' messages on the fag packets.)

But when depression, cancer of the mind, kills somebody, that is, they kill themselves,

"Suddenly ……." "Without warning,"

It would not be seen as an ending to a courageous struggle. Neither would it be seen as a dignified way out of overwhelming torment and sorrow. HOWEVER! Unlike the lung cancer induced by smoking, the depression could well have been induced by circumstances beyond the person's control! A chemical imbalance in the brain is no more the fault of the sufferer than epilepsy or catching a cold! Childhood abuse is not the child's fault either, but by golly they suffer for it, often with depression in later years! Do you see what I'm trying to say here? If we dare to attach a stigma to suicide, that is, untimely death, then we need to have a massive rethink and overhaul our entire attitude to mental health issues.

Suicide is seen as the ultimate selfish act. (Is smoking???? Is being obese?) I have tried to kill myself. Whether that was seen as a real attempt or a cry for attention I don't know and I truly don't care. I meant to do it. I knew all the gut wrenching arguments about motherless kids. I argued with my psychiatrist until I ran out of words, but such was my pain at the time that I believed with all my heart that they would be better off without me and I would be doing them a massive favour. I still believe that.

After my failed suicide attempt nobody was told what was wrong with me when I spent the next few days in bed, drowsy, sleeping, retching and vomiting. Frank looked after me and cried with me and despaired of any lasting solution to the bloody miserable existence that was mine. A secret and lonely malady. And a sad one.

"Self pitying bitch!"   Yeh!   SO WHAT?????

THE HUDDLE

CHAPTER FIVE   FEELING A BIT ANGRY

I am now feeling angry about them. The Huddle. But this time, instead of smashing a dish, doing vigorous aerobic exercise or falling into a self pitying depression, I am going to try and type the anger out of me by attempting to explain exactly what The Huddle make me angry about! In doing so I shall try not to use their language as I don't want to lower myself to their pathetic, miserable level. I am low enough as it is. How *dare* they blaspheme and carry on a string of obscenities, filling my ears with their filth and disgusting language! I've quoted some of it for the purpose of illustrating just what this voice hearer hears. Even then I use *s to try and soften the blow for any reader! How thoughtful of me!

The Huddle! What the hell are they anyway? Satan's little minions! That's all. Their obsequiousness, their crawling servitude to him has to be experienced to be believed. They make themselves out to be so darn big and powerful and strong, but they are nothing but his pathetic, easy for God to trample on, little minions!! So why doesn't God trample on them! Come on, God! Why not?

Does God hate me or not want me that he should allow these THINGS to shadow and taint and spoil my life? Is God angry with The Huddle? Is it something very wrong about me that keeps The Huddle with me? Am I an unforgiven category 'A' sinner?

Damn The Huddle to the lowest depths of hell and beyond! Destroy them and damn them! Dr.

Kapp keeps on about being almost sorry for their pathetic existence and being able to lovingly commit them to God for Him to deal with in whatever way He sees fit. Like I was able to do with my evil comforter. But I liked and wanted my evil comforter! I could not see that he was harming or controlling my life! The Huddle are different. I don't curl up on a chair and enjoy listening to them. I cannot truly feel sorry for them. Sometimes I will say that I almost do, but I am then only trying to please my psychiatrist. It is very difficult to have feelings other then anger and hatred at them for the way in which they darken my existence. I won't call it my life.

THEY ARE DRIVING ME NUTS AND I AM ABSOLUTELY BLOODY SICK OF THEM!!!!!!!!!!!!!!!!!!!!!!!!!!!!!!!!!!!!!

I go to bed and the last words I hear are "Bitch is going to sleep now." However many times I wake up during the night, the first words I hear are "Bitch is awake!" There is not one part of my stupid, useless existence that they do not infiltrate, affect, comment upon, laugh about, hate or spoil. Et cetera. They are invasive unwelcome usurpers. Incompatible with a happy, productive and peaceful life. The Huddle?...

DAMN THEM TO HELL!!!!!!!!!!!!!!!!!!!!!!!!!!!!!!!!!

They are very angry with me now for typing all this. I know perfectly well what will happen next if I carry on ignoring their commands to stop typing,

THE HUDDLE

which I am so far managing to do. They will send the worms to come wriggling up through the typewriter keys. Worms that I cannot feel, but can see winding themselves around my fingers, obliterating the typewriter keys ... They have sent worms before and I've abandoned my typewriter for months, too scared to use it. Therefore a victory for The Huddle.

But rest assured, cruel voices, that if the worms happen again and I can't see what I'm typing, then I shall write about you instead. It'll take longer, but that doesn't matter. Either way I WILL finish this book! I'm used to being frightened senseless by you, I know what you're like. Maybe it's time to develop a little more immunity to your cruel and nasty attacks.

Don't you **DARE** hurt or frighten me. Just DON'T!!

"So what'll YOU f**king do about it then BITCH?"

Do you know that I'm not allowed to wear anything white? That's because white stands for purity, virginity and the state of being unspoiled, and I am, apparently, a father f**ker, a whore and a slut. Last summer I bought myself a lovely white t-shirt and did manage to wear it a few times. Stood in my bedroom I would put it on, then take it straight back off because The Huddle were at me about it. Then I would come over all strong and decide to ignore them and put the t-shirt back on again. Then I would take it back off! Eventually I would get the hang of tuning out of The Huddle for long enough to put the t-shirt on, leave it on, and wear it for a few hours. Sound silly? Try it one morning. Ask your nearest and dearest to tell you that what you're wearing is wrong for you. It looks dreadful, makes you look fatter, not for you, does absolutely nothing for you, etc.. Wouldn't that make you want to get changed? – Especially if they were going to keep on moaning about it for hours and hours?

My favourite blouse happens to be one of those pretty, frilly jobs from Laura Ashley (bought in mint condition from a charity shop for a couple of quid! Absolute bargain!!) It is also white. So. Same problem! I put it on – eventually – then spend half a day hearing The Huddle telling me to take it off! I am a f**king slut and too dirty and satanic to wear it. (So much for not lowering myself to write their language eh?)

Ignoring The Huddle and telling them to shove off would seem like sensible, obvious advice. In fact, so blasted obvious that it doesn't need to be given! Of course I've told them to shove off, and worse. It doesn't work. If it did, I wouldn't have them and I'll bet most other voice hearers wouldn't have their nasty voices either.

Both Frank and Dr. Kapp exhort me to tell The Huddle to get lost and I am apt to accept their no doubt well meaning advice as cruel and not a little patronising. Do they think I don't make every effort to ignore this wretched Huddle? Do they think I never tell them to get lost? If Joe Bloggs had boils on his bum would they disappear if he told them to get lost, shove off and get the hell out of his life?? Doubtful. Poor old Joe would either have to learn to live with his boils, like I'm learning to live with The

THE HUDDLE

Huddle, or else have them excised (like I was exorcised), or else suffer until they maybe go of their own accord, like I'm hoping The Huddle will one day soon. Disappear!

Maybe some blessed winged creature will zoom down from heaven, put hands upon my head, and welcome me into the fold of God, thus delivering me from The Huddle. Will I only be free of them when I am dead? Will I now have to accept that I have them and go ahead learning a little better how to cope with them? But why should I accept something that is so evil and against God? Surely that's not the right thing to do?

Advice to ignore them and tell them to shove off is bloody cruel and given in total damn ignorance of what the experience of hearing voices is like!! That's how I feel. That's part of the reason I'm writing this book!! Ridiculous, stupid advice – shouldn't even be called advice! Sorry Frank. Sorry Dr. Kapp. You've both done a whoopsie on this one! (And I'm not really sorry either – I mean it sarcastically.)

Have you ever noticed that 'Santa' is an anagram of 'Satan'?

"Who is it that comes to bitch witch at Christmas and…"

O SHOVE OFF!!!!!!!!!!!

Even while I sleep I'm not free of them. They sneak into my dreams and make themselves mnemonics of my past. They frighten me, they wake me up, they laugh at me from their place in the window and then they drive me out of my warm and cosy bed. So don't get up, I hear you say. Ignore them! Well, I've already told you off about that train of thought. Remember I'm the expert here! You have them for a day and ignore them! I manage to do an awful lot of ignoring. If I didn't I would have been cut to ribbons and dead years ago.

So they wake me up and follow me down the stairs before jumping into the butterfly, desk lamp, television or, recently, an ornament I have on the coffee table. And yes, I have thought about putting this ornament away, but I know, and you know, that it wouldn't work. If they seek a new home in my living room then they will find one, however much stuff I move, hide, or get rid of. Other than living a totally minimalist life (how boring) there is nothing I can do about this.

Rachel lives in a bare cell. Bare walls, no furniture, no anything. And Rachel still hears voices. Voices do not necessarily have to come *from* something, but if they chose to do so, then there's not a lot you can do about it. In fact I would go as far as to say there is *nothing* you can do about it!

Next? The bathroom! I am so very angry, frustrated, sick and tired of having no privacy in the bathroom. It's disgusting! I wish The Huddle would not be there, gawping at me, sniggering, and providing an obscene, filthy accompaniment to my daily ablutions. Telling me to pick up my own s**t and eat it, lick the toilet, suck a used sanitary towel, pee in a tooth mug and drink it. Et cetera!

THE HUDDLE

I wish I could have a shower in peace without them hating my ugly body and accusing me of sexually abusing myself as I wash. They threaten to jump into the shower head and then rain down upon me as blood. Sometimes I've seen blood coming out of the shower head, but it isn't blood! It's only ever water! I have to keep reassuring myself about that.

I very rarely have a bath these days. That's partly because our bath taps need replacing and it takes ages for the bath to fill, and partly because The Huddle will jump into the taps and threaten to scald my feet and/or turn the bathwater into blood or liquid filth. Sometimes they will jump into a bar of soap, and so I keep two bars in the bathroom so that I can wash with the Huddle free soap.

I am angry because I can't even go shopping without them following me up and down the aisles of the supermarket. Tomato sauce is bottled blood, Rice Krispies are maggots, sausages are penises, and tins of biscuits contain dead foetuses. Et cetera. Want me to go on? Yogurt is seminal fluid, lemonade is urine, chocolate biscuits are covered in s**t……. Get the picture?

When I reach the checkout The Huddle leave the space around my head and jump into somewhere else. If I'm shopping in Asda then they will jump into the light above checkout number nineteen, and if I'm at Tesco they'll jump into one of the two saving stamp machines situated opposite the checkouts. I have to buy my stamps from the Huddle free machine, quickly, before they transfer into the one I'm feeding money to. I would not like that. Feeding them money. They already take too much from me. Enough is enough!

Are you by now maybe wondering how I live without being totally psychotic and needing permanent incarceration in a mental institution? Well, if I was to be mad, then what would my madness be other than a manifestation of intolerable mental torment? Or perhaps I really *am* mad! My madness being that I *do* appear to be leading a normal sort of life, putting up with it and coping with it. Maybe the people we call 'mad' are more normal than the rest of us because their minds refuse to tolerate the intolerable. Again I ask, what is normality anyway?

I have just looked up the word 'madness' in my friend the dictionary. (See? I do have a friend after all!) It says,

Insanity, lunacy.

Extreme anger, excitement or foolishness.

I *am* bloody well mad then! I am extremely angry! Mad with them. Mad with myself. Mad with you, dear reader. Mad with you because you don't hear The Huddle and I'm trying to tell you what it's like and I'm very frustrated because I don't think I'm clever enough to convey my experiences lucidly or expertly. Damn them! Damn you! Damn me!

The Huddle are mad, round the twist, and a bunch of pathetic lunatics. Why else would they keep on the way they do? What a pathetic existence, sent to torment little old me from dawn till dusk and in between. How absolutely pathetic. What a complete waste of their time and my time. They are nothing but lousy bloody time wasters!

THE HUDDLE

Just think of what I could be doing instead of wasting my time employing a variety of coping mechanisms in order to continue as normal a life, or existence, as possible.

The Huddle are also incredibly boring. They say the same thing and pass the same comments over and over and over again, day after day after day, week after week after week, year after year after bloody year. What a way to exist! For goodness sake, don't they get bored and fed up with *themselves*? Do they hate what they do? They certainly don't seem to, always taking great delight in their career of torment and humiliation. Cruel spoilers! Foul and evil LITTLE minions!!!

DAMN THEM TO HELL!!!!!!!!!!!!!!!!!!!!!!!!!!!!

Did you notice earlier on in this chapter that I referred to a dictionary as my friend? You did? Clever! Your concentration is obviously a lot better than mine. When I read I frequently have to re-read sentences and paragraphs because I've lost the gist of what I'm reading. I know loads of people do this, but I'd prefer the losing of the gist to be due to thoughts of what's for dinner, or thinking about the kids, or the shopping list, or *any* gist pincher rather than the activity of The Huddle. That's why a dictionary has become a friend! At times I read that instead of a book as there is no story line to spoil or interrupt, no sentences or paragraphs, just lots of words and their meanings. I love to look at words! Hence my dictionary is another coping mechanism when even the Woman's Own is not accessible to me.

Janet Cooper

I can get exceptionally angry in the kitchen where they can provoke me so much that I will hurl a plate or dish across the room and cringe as it shatters against the back door. How wonderful it would be to mix a 'Mummy Special' chocolate cake without being told I'm mixing diarrhoea or liquid s**t! Fruit jelly is angel vomit, soup is sick ... I don't need to go on, I'm sure you are good at getting the picture by now.

Food is an awkward issue with The Huddle around, although I do concede that my history of anorexia is no doubt contributory to my issues with food. At the moment I'm only 'allowed' to eat toast, fruit and yogurt. It's been this way for a very long time although I do indulge in the occasional small slice of cake, crisp (singular), small biccy or ultra small slice of pizza.

"Not allowed to eat that! Fat f**king slut ... Don't you DARE eat that! ... Fat pig; see what glutton stuffs in her fat frigging mouth..."

Some days I have to force myself to eat even the foods I'm allowed. I do not want to lose weight because then I would lose my job again, and below seven stone I become lethargic, weak, shaky and my periods stop. Jan could not work when we were like that, and the job was given up for eighteen months. That must not happen again.

Anorexia was one of my more destructive coping mechanisms and I do not consider myself anywhere near cured of it. I'm a recovering anorexic! Like an alcoholic! Once an alcoholic, always an alcoholic. Once an anorexic, always an

THE HUDDLE

anorexic. Don't have that one drink. Don't skip that first meal.

Where was I? Oh yes, in the kitchen. Here The Huddle come from the taps or the kettle. My kettle doesn't sing, it talks! Ha ha, very funny! I scoop Persil into a measuring cup,

"You f**king need stain digesters, you filthy…"

and they tell me that the powder is really maggots and I am pouring maggots into the washing machine. They would very much like me to put my head in the microwave and frizzle it to hell on full power while they hoot with laughter. Or else I could plunge my head into the washing up water and drown. They command me to burn myself on the cooker and pour the contents of the rubbish bag over myselves. My*self*. I am told to eat cat food and drink bleach. Always, always, always, always when I am in the kitchen The Huddle tell me to cut myself and kill us. I almost hear the tablets in the cupboard calling out to be swallowed in a fatal overdose. How I wish …

When my body has been cut, if it is one of my other personalities who has done it, then I will have no memory of the act whatsoever. If it has been done by Katy, I will 'come round' to find myself in a mess, covered in blood and often still holding a knife. If it has been Rachel then I will find myself already cleaned up, a bloodied towel might be soaking in the sink and some sort of dressing covering the wound. I will then check to see if the wound needs suturing. If not too deep, I'll apply steri-strips and care for it myself.

There have been times, however, when I have deliberately cut myself. Sometimes simply because they have told me to do it and I've done it! Sometimes, I'm ashamed to say, after a degree of planning. I have justified this self mutilation as a way of punishing myself for having The Huddle and therefore being the awful person that I am. I have seen it as a symbolic way of letting the badness out of me and getting rid of it, rather like a profuse flow of blood cleanses germs and debris from out of a wound. I do not feel pain when I cut myself, even though many of the cuts have been very deep and on one occasion the casualty doctor was unable to suture my arm and had to call in a Consultant to do it, I'd done such a 'good' job!

Knowing the pain and discomfort I experience for many days, sometimes weeks, following suturing, I came to see this physical suffering as yet another coping mechanism; focusing on the pain to keep The Huddle in the background. After a cut is made the relief is incredible; almost euphoric as all those little endorphins rush to my brain cells. There is something perversely thrilling to see the blood pooling in a deep slice before spilling over and running away; I've let something out, released something, Yet like my anorexia it is a destructive, negative coping mechanism and one I am now pleased I've been able to give up, although at times I would still like to do it. Having The Huddle constantly encouraging me in this direction does not exactly help me!

So you see, I do ignore them quite a bit, don't I! I told you that I wanted this account to be an encouragement to me, so I'm encouraging myself

THE HUDDLE

and being encouraged! I *am* able to ignore them. Lots of times I *do* ignore them. So there!

I have just eaten my lunch; a slice of toast and a small banana. Pretty safe food. It was allowed. So are you ready now to hear a bit more of what I spend a lot of time trying to ignore? Be warned that it won't make pleasant reading, my apologies, but you can always skip a few pages if it offends. I wish it was that easy for me to get away from it!

The Huddle! They humiliate me and want to see me humiliated. No wonder I get to feel so angry about them, and what they persist in telling me, commanding me, to do. They tell me, command me, to smell my pants when I go to the loo, look at dog s**t, pick it up and eat it, put my finger inside my vagina and lick it, make myself sick and eat it, destroy things in the house, cut myself, kill myself, kill my family, kill the pets, exorcise myself, suck my own nipples, lick the cat's a*se, expose myself, masturbate, imagine other people masturbating, kill my mother, smash dishes, set fire to the house, set fire to churches, destroy my bible, rip out the pages and use them as loo paper, cut up my clothes, everybody hates me, God hates me and the whole of bloody heaven hates me!

This is a very small example of The Huddle on a normal, not so bad day, like today. This is a pretty good day because I have been able to keep myself busy without resorting to drugging myself up and sleeping in a chair to waste time until I'm dead. It is a good day because I feel a little in control and tuned out of The Huddle. They have not been unbearably bad and worms have not yet oozed out of my typewriter. It is a good day because I haven't killed the cat, drunk urine, sicked up my lunch, ripped up this book, prayed to the devil, smashed my head against a wall, cut myself, throttled the desk lamp or taken a fatal overdose. It is indeed a wonderful day! I have ignored so much!! Aren't I clever?

But will somebody please help me? You! Husband who lives with me. You! Psychiatrist with a magic wand! Because I don't know how long I can keep up the being alright. I have recently stopped taking my medication and am missing some of its effects, though I know that I'm not as depressed as I have been or could be, and that is good and relieving. I am not mad or ill or sick in the head; I just have the others and The Huddle. That's all. And this *is* a good day!

"Tell the damn truth, Janet!" (This is me speaking here!)

Even on a good day I am s**t scared most of the time and on the verge of panic. What am I frightened of? Lots of stuff! Like the voices getting worse so that I am no longer able to function adequately. Going into St. Cadoc's again. Killing myself. I am frightened of failing at suicide and waking up in hospital. I am frightened of God. I am frightened of Satan. I am frightened of The Huddle. I am frightened of Dr. Kapp disappearing before I feel able to cope without her visits. I am frightened of anger, hatred, violence, swearing and threats – as uttered by The Huddle or other people. I am frightened of my mind becoming as sick and

THE HUDDLE

perverted as the voices it hears. My mind. I am frightened for my mind.

Is it all going to get worse instead of better? No more now. Please, no more. Rest the typewriter, for it is tired. But no! There is no rest! They tell me to sick my whole s**t self up and roll in my own vomit. They tell me to s**t on the carpet, s**t on the piano keys, straddle the cat and p*ss on her f**king head, all the while pretending it's somebody else's head. They tell me to hit myself, either with my hands or with an implement. They tell me to hide s**t in the beds, hack off Frank's penis and either eat it, feed it to the cat or cook it for tea! If that sounds the slightest bit funny, then believe me, it isn't. I'm definitely not laughing! I could go on and on and on and on and on, but I need to have a break here because I'm crying and finding it hard to see through the tears…

"Shame!!" Huddle laughter…

It is later in the day now. My children are home from school, have had their tea and are busy doing homework with friends. My beautiful daughter handed me an essay she had begun to write but did not feel able to go on with. My daughter is ten. This is what she wrote:

My Mum's Voices

The Huddle, what they say is, "I'll stick my tongue out at her I'll shout I'll spit I'll say rude words."

It made me feel so sad. My children know about The Huddle. As much as they are capable of knowing and understanding at ages ten and twelve. They will also tell me that I should shout at the voices to shove off and go away. I accept their advice with so much more grace than I do when it is given by Frank or my psychiatrist. Ah well…

Another thing which makes me angry with The Huddle, although in this case my hopelessness at the situation far outweighs my anger, is the way that they accuse me. Accusers of the brethren! The Bible says; yet having been banned from attending (Reverend H's) church I do not feel I qualify as one of God's brethren! Even when I am doing something that is normal and good and okay then they will still accuse me, making me feel I'm not good at anything and everything I do is wrong. Category 'A' sinner. God's reject. Unforgiven witch. Satan's little puppet. But their worst accusations come when they have goaded me into doing something and I have given in and done it. For example, if they have spent seven hours goading me to cut myself and I've eventually given in to them and carried out the act, then they will immediately cease their goading and start accusing me of doing the very thing that they set out to make me do in the first place!

"Oooooooh! Look what the stupid bitch has gone and done now … What she do that for? She's in deep trouble … Wait till her f**king husband finds out … You s*dding well gone and done it now, girlie!"

THE HUDDLE

See what I mean! Boy! Would they have a field day! It is *so* infuriating! Frank would arrive home from work to find me nursing yet another sutured wound and would rant and rave, despairing at the bizarre situation and shouting at me, much to The Huddle's amusement and alongside their continuing accusations.

At his wits end with me one day, Frank rang St. Cadoc's hospital and spoke to a consultant I had once seen there. What was this psychiatrist's patronising, cruel and ignorant suggestion?

"Maybe your wife should get a job Mr. Cooper!"

I had a job!! What the hell did this arrogant jerk think I was? Some bored housewife who had nothing better to do than cut herself with knives? I HAVE A BLOODY JOB YOU IGNORANT, CRUEL PIG!!!!!! I've lost count of the number of times I've struggled to get Jan into work, in pain from my wounds, watching while she spends each shift secretly swallowing Paracetamol and checking that blood has not oozed out and stained her uniform.

We kept a very painful secret, Jan and I. On one occasion Jan went into work only hours after I'd had twenty stitches in my arm and sixteen across my chest. I don't know how she got through that ten hour shift.

So there! I have a job. I don't find it easy but at least I do make the effort and manage to work twenty, thirty, even forty hours a week. How I wish I had the time and the peace and quiet to be bored!

So, Mr. Clever Consultant, don't you DARE go telling Frank that maybe I just need to get a job!

Maybe **_you_** need to get a job! Out of psychiatry! You weren't particularly understanding for a SHRINK, were you? Perhaps I should send you this book to read. Good idea! I'll send one to all your shrinky, arrogant colleagues as well. You must be one of the ones who opted for psychiatry because you didn't make the grade anywhere else, and kept forgetting which side of the body the appendix lies!!

Notice how I've turned from being angry with The Huddle to being angry with a psychiatrist? I think the mind doctors call that transference or something. It's The Huddle I'm supposed to be angry with in this chapter, not some doctor quack who knew too little about me to be making such cruel and hurtful insinuations and suggestions. But that's how it goes. That's the sort of thing that happens. If The Huddle had not incited me to self mutilate then Frank wouldn't have made that phone call. Ridiculously I am still incredibly hurt by that consultant's words. He hurt me. How DARE another human being hurt me AGAIN!!!!! It's not fair.

"Self pitying bitch!"

Yes, indeed I am.

So you see, I am not only angry with The Huddle, I feel anger towards other people as well, and probably not always with justification. I'm angry with Frank because he doesn't hear voices and can be short tempered with me. I also become extremely angry with him for always telling me that

THE HUDDLE

one day I will be rid of The Huddle. How does he know? What if I never am? Will he still love me? If they never go, then I shall have let him down and become a massive disappointment to him as he is so positive about their eventual departure. Maybe he is comforting himself by constantly saying this – it certainly isn't comforting me!! I have just about given up hope. (Have I …?)

I also feel anger towards my psychiatrist because she doesn't hear voices either. I get even angrier when she tells me that I am angry! For a long time I absolutely refused to admit to feeling or being angry. (That was following my counselling with Reverend H. who told me that my anger was sin and ordered me to repent.) I get angry about some of the things Dr. Kapp says to me, even if she means them for my eventual good. I feel especially angry towards other psychiatrists I have seen in the past. Don't know why. Or maybe I do? Perhaps it's because they haven't helped me; they haven't talked to me and tried to understand me, and they had barely listened to me.

I get angry with this one shop assistant in my local Spar because she slams my change down and never speaks to me or looks at me. I feel angry towards so many people from my past, be they dead or alive. I get angry with myself, angry with Jan and Rachel and Liz and Katy and Janny. I get angry with Satan. Most of all I get angry with God because He has the power to heal but does not. Is it because of my past sins that He refuses to take The Huddle from me? Why does he refuse to heal other, more deserving people?

Lord, "Hear me, lest otherwise they should rejoice over me: when my foot slippeth they magnify themselves against me. For I am ready to halt, and my sorrow is continually before me. For I will declare my iniquity. I will be sorry for my sins. But mine enemies are lively and they are strong." (Psalm38:16-19) The Huddle. My enemy.

"The Lord shall swallow them up in His wrath, and the fire shall devour them." (Psalm 20:9) But the Lord *doesn't* swallow them up in anger, and fire does not destroy them! I wish I could say this to God – "Thou hast also given me the shield of thy salvation; and thy right hand hath holden me up, and thy gentleness hath made me great. Thou hast enlarged my steps under me that my feet did not slip. I have pursued mine enemies, and overtaken them: Neither did I turn again until they were consumed. I have wounded them that they are not able to rise: they are fallen under my feet. For thou hast girded me with strength unto the battle: thou hast subdued under me those that rose up against me. Thou hast also given me the necks of my enemies; that I might destroy them that hate me. They cried, but there was none to save them: even unto the Lord, but He answered them not. Then did I beat them small as the dust before the wind; I did cast them out as dirt in the streets." (Psalm 18:35-42)

Instead, this would seem more appropriate – "My God, my God, why hast thou forsaken me? Why art thou so far off from helping me, and from the words of my roaring? O my God, I cry in the daytime but thou hearest not; and in the night season, and am not silent. All that see me laugh

THE HUDDLE

me to scorn: they shoot out the lip, they shake the head, saying, he trusted on the Lord that He would deliver him. They gaped upon me with their mouths, as a ravening and roaring lion. … the assembly of the wicked have enclosed me." (Psalm 22) Does God forget that The Huddle is His enemy also?

Another verse of scripture tells me, "All thine enemies have opened their mouths against thee: they hiss and gnash the teeth: they say, we have swallowed her up." (Lamentations 2:16) Then in the next chapter of the book of Lamentations it says that God does not afflict willingly. So why *does* He do it then? Why God? WHY??? Lord, WHY!!!?? Why me? Why anybody?

JUST WHY????????

I am angry with You! So angry!!

"Mine eye trickleth down and ceaseth not… Mine enemies chased me sore … Thou hast seen all their vengeance and their imaginations against me; the lips of those that rose up against me, and their devices against me all the day… I am their music… Persecute and destroy them in anger from under the heavens…"

I am also angry with God because I have come to love Jesus. Does that make any sense? Maybe not. I say that I love Jesus and The Huddle say that I don't, cannot possibly, and never will. Jesus does not want me to love Him and they say my love is a satanic delusion. But why does loving Jesus create such a battle within me? It is supposed to bring joy and peace and the knowledge of sins forgiven.

Instead I feel as if I've been chucked on a battle field. The Huddle against Jesus – God against Satan. I have the battle scars on my body. Come and take a look at them! They're not pretty.

It is a battle for me to send up any sort of prayer. It is a battle to read the beautiful and sometimes not so beautiful scriptures. It is a battle to sing a hymn. I realise and I surely know that Jesus is everything that The Huddle is not, and never could be. He is good and pure and gentle and lovely. Oh! The absolute purity of Jesus! How it clashes with the darkness in my mind! How utterly beautiful is the light of Christ! Jesus is sinless, He is safe to be with, He loves me, He will never hurt me, O God why did You see Him murdered on a cross? How could you? I am so angry with You!!

I know how wonderful Jesus is and I know how awful The Huddle are. A taste of heaven and a taste of hell, all mixed up inside me and I am in agony. I cannot bear it. I hear the cross and I cannot bear the pain of it.

"…whatsoever things are pure, whatsoever things are lovely, whatsoever things are of good report … think on these things." (Philippians 4:8) Beautiful, beautiful words but … "F**k the bast**d Christ and suck up sweet angel puke …" It is so very opposite and I am in agony. Take the first line of a hymn – "O worship the Lord in the beauty of holiness." How can I? There is no beauty or holiness in my life! Nothing lovely about me to bring me closer to Jesus. Just The Huddle; the total opposite of the truth and the loveliness and the beauty and the gentleness of Jesus my saviour.

THE HUDDLE

Rachel used to hate God, being angry with Him and swearing at Him. Amazingly, however, she has turned a full circle and displays a love and a trust towards Jesus of which I am envious. She prays. Little words in little sentences – all very childish, but that doesn't matter. We have to be as little children in order to know the Kingdom of heaven. Yes. Rachel also loves Jesus. How wonderful!

It is a delight to me that I do not feel anger towards my children. Of course I get annoyed with them at times, the same as any other Mum, but it is not the sort of anger I've been talking about here. It's not the sort of anger that gnarls you up inside and makes you hate people. I just feel very sorry for my children because they have me for a mother. I bet you, dear reader, are also feeling sorry for them by now. That's sad.

Anger can also be useful to me, enabling me to continue my daily struggle with The Huddle. If I lost all my anger towards them then they would indeed swallow me up. You need to have anger towards an enemy in order to fight against them in a battle.

This is something I wrote when very depressed and *not* feeling angry with the Huddle! I had stopped coping with them.

JANET'S DEAD!

Janet is no longer alive
But passed over into a living death,
With evil breath,
A spirit of depression.
As such she hovers just outside this body,
Watching it perform its daily chores

Janet Cooper

With regular monotony.

Evil spirit of depression
Sees the body, heavy and unwilling,
Any task fulfilling
Is such gigantic effort.
Hard and slow.
Limbs don't want to go.

O please! Please leave us all alone!
Life! You are not wanted.
We command you now with all our strength to
Leave!! Please leave and let all here be dead.

For voices in this head
Go on and on and on and on …
Chlorpromazine dulls reception,
Nothing more.
They still are there to swear and mock
And say to kill.
O heart, all here do beg thee,
Stop thy evil beating
And be still.
Dead.
All dead!
Please!!!
We beg and beg and long and wish and soon must do.
Be dead.

But once again, today, the pills have taken over,
Sleeping, dreaming, trip a torture nightmare
In a field of evil clover,
While they mutter on in thickest grass,

THE HUDDLE

"That's right, that's right, go on, go on,
Don't die until tomorrow.
Go take a pill instead!
Chemical relief for poorly head
Until you shall be dead."

Chlorpromazine dulls reception.
They don't go.
Chlorpromazine dulls reception.
Nothing then
Except indifference and depression.
Nothing. Nothing.
Janet is now nothing.
Janet's dead!

"Lord, how long shall the wicked triumph? How long shall they utter and speak hard things? Who will rise up for me against the evil doers? Or who will stand up for me against the workers of iniquity? And he shall bring upon them their own iniquity, and shall cut them off in their own wickedness; yea, the Lord our God shall cut them off." (Psalm 94) "For mine enemies speak against me: and they that lay wait for my soul take counsel together, saying, God hath forsaken (her): for there is none to deliver (her). O God, be not far from me: O my God, make haste for my help. Let them be confounded and consumed that are adversaries to my soul; let them be covered with reproach and dishonour that seek my hurt." (Psalm 71) "I will say unto God my rock, why hast thou forgotten me; while they say daily, where is thy God?" (Psalm 42)

Yes. I am so very angry with God. In Isaiah it says, "The wicked are like the troubled sea, when it cannot rest, whose waters cast up mire and dirt. There is no peace, sayeth God, to the wicked." (Isaiah 57:20,21) Don't you think this is a good description of The Huddle? They *are* troubled. They *cannot* rest. They keep churning up muck and filth. They themselves know no peace.

Why, then, does God *not* deal with them? Why not, God? Why not?? Do You hate *me*? Are *You* angry with *me*?

For Christ's sake, help me!! Take them away from me, heal my mind, calm and soothe me, be gentle with me for I hurt so much.

LOVE ME!!!!!!!! Lord, what is it about me that keeps me separate from you? What have I done? What have I not confessed and sorrowed over? Is it because of my unforgiveness? If so, then tell me please, show me please, help me please ……..

HOW DO I FORGIVE A RAPIST???????????????

DAMN WELL TELL ME HOW TO!!!!!!!!!!!!!!!!!!!!!!!!!!

Are other things about me, most things, so wrong and *so* unforgiven? I cry bitter tears and my very soul undergoes periods of rot and decay, I hear His cross and I am in agony. The Huddle pick on me and torment me daily. My nights are battles. Why, God, is there no peace and no relief? How do I continue to offend You?

Then forgive me! A thousand times forgive me and make me truly sorry for my sin. Heal my mind and give me peace. Please!! I am frightened for the

THE HUDDLE

mind I share with those I share it with. The voices will surely drive us crazy. Did You not see me the other night? You who sees all? How we paced up and down the living room like a tormented animal, hands clapped tight over my ears in a bid to shut them out of our head? Hot tears, so many of them, rolled down fat cheeks that night. The rest of my family slept peacefully. I was in agony! WHAT have I done wrong? WHAT am I doing wrong that I should continue to be this way? What is wrong with us? Maybe we should not be.

God? I desire that You should speak to me these words. "For a small moment I have forsaken thee; but with great mercies I will gather thee. In a little wrath I hid my face from thee for a moment; but with everlasting kindness will I have mercy on thee, saith the Lord thy redeemer. O thou afflicted, tossed with tempest and not comforted … all thy children shall be taught of the Lord; and great shall be the peace of thy children. In righteousness …

"She still quote f**king sweet f**king scripture whipped her, rubbish boring rubbish boring rubbish f**k muck f**k muck…"

Yes. I am going to keep quoting scripture! I believe it's relevant to my state, and it's MY book anyway.

"…In righteousness shalt thou be established; thou shalt be far from oppression; for thou shalt not fear; and from terror; for it shall not come near thee. … Whosoever shall gather against thee shall fall for thy sake. (Isaiah 54) For ye shall go out with joy, and be led forth with peace: The mountains and the hills shall break forth before you with singing, and all the trees of the field shall clap their hands." (Isaiah 55)

Beautiful, beautiful words.........

I was angry yesterday evening. Why? Well, do you know what Frank said to me? And on a day when I was rather pleased with how I'd managed to get through each hour. He told me I was totally frazzled and looked as if I had forks of lightening zooming out from all over me!! And there was me thinking I was pretty okay.
"You're not okay, love, you're nowhere near okay!"
Thanks a bundle! I do love a bit of positive encouragement and kind words!
So, well, alright then, it hadn't been a particularly brilliant day as The Huddle had been quite bad, or perhaps my reception of them was somewhat more acute, and I'd had to fight the temptation to reach for the little white pills to calm everything down. Rachel'd had one of her crying sessions and little Janny was making those irritatingly sad little crying, moaning noises. But when Frank had passed his comment that I was nowhere near okay, he was sat at the table eating his meat, three veg. and gravy dinner which had been placed before him within minutes of his arrival home from work. The house was warm and tidy. I'd tidied round, cleaned the kids rooms (well, the bits that you could see!), done the vacuuming, made the beds, the washing and ironing was up to date, the kids welcomed home from school and fed, a trolley load of shopping had

THE HUDDLE

been got from the supermarket, I'd managed a bit of this typing, and the cat had had her munchies!! I'd done all this after a ten hour night shift after which I'd only slept for two hours in the morning!

WHAT THE HELL DOES HE EXPECT ME TO BE LIKE WHEN I _AM_ OKAY??? BLOODY SUPERWOMAN??????????

Yes, I know, I know, I'm being silly. Or am I? Of course, being constantly on the go is one of my better coping mechanisms but it is an exhausting one. Frank meant that I was jittery, bothered a lot by The Huddle and not feeling brilliant. But I'd coped alright! What the hell else can I damn well bloody do? I'm sick of it but I can't get rid of it.

Damn this miserable existence! I should bloody well never have been bloody well born! Don't bother to excuse my language! The tears, the ones I refuse to shed, form a lake within me and we are slowly drowning in it. Down and down and down. Deeper and deeper and deeper. Almost, almost, almost at the bottom, then Angel will drag me back up again and again and again. Maybe there are seconds when I know Jesus. Just seconds. Then heaven disappears again and once more I am sharing hell and I cope for a bit longer. Somehow. Because I have no choice.

The battle is long and hard and angry. It is not yet won, which means *I* have not yet *lost*. But who will eventually claim the victory?

Lord, deliver me from the anger that is wrong and destructive, the anger on which The Huddle feed, the anger that is against You. Instead, make me peaceful and give me silence. Make me gentle and holy. Make me loving, help me to love, for "Love is patient, love is kind. It does not envy, it does not boast, it is not proud. It is not rude, it is not self seeking, it is not easily angered, it keeps no record of wrongs. Love does not delight in evil but rejoices with the truth. It always protects, always trusts, always hopes, always perseveres." (1Corinthians 13:4-7) How beautiful! How opposite to The Huddle. Lord, keep me opposite to them!!

I must close this chapter now. Are you wondering about the worms that live in my typewriter? Did The Huddle force them up between the keys to squirm all around my fingers? Yes, they did. It's one of their more regular tricks which I find hard to blot from my mind and cope with. The trouble is, it happened so often in the past, resulting in a *bad* reaction from me, that they can't resist trying it again and again, and I can't stop expecting it to happen again and again. And yes, the last time it happened I *did* jump up, frightened, and burst into tears, slamming the lid back on the typewriter. Wouldn't you? But I eventually came back and carried on typing. Would you? My reaction hadn't been *quite* violent enough to reduce The Huddle to a loud state of demonic hilarity. So they did give up. It isn't very nice though.

"Self pity, bitch is s**tty. Self pitying holy cow...."

Yeh. I am. So what?

Want to know *when* the worms came? It was when I was quoting all that scripture a few pages

THE HUDDLE

back. "For their worm shall not die, neither shall their fire be quenched; and they shall be an abhorring to all flesh." (Isaiah 66:24)

Goodnight!

Janet Cooper

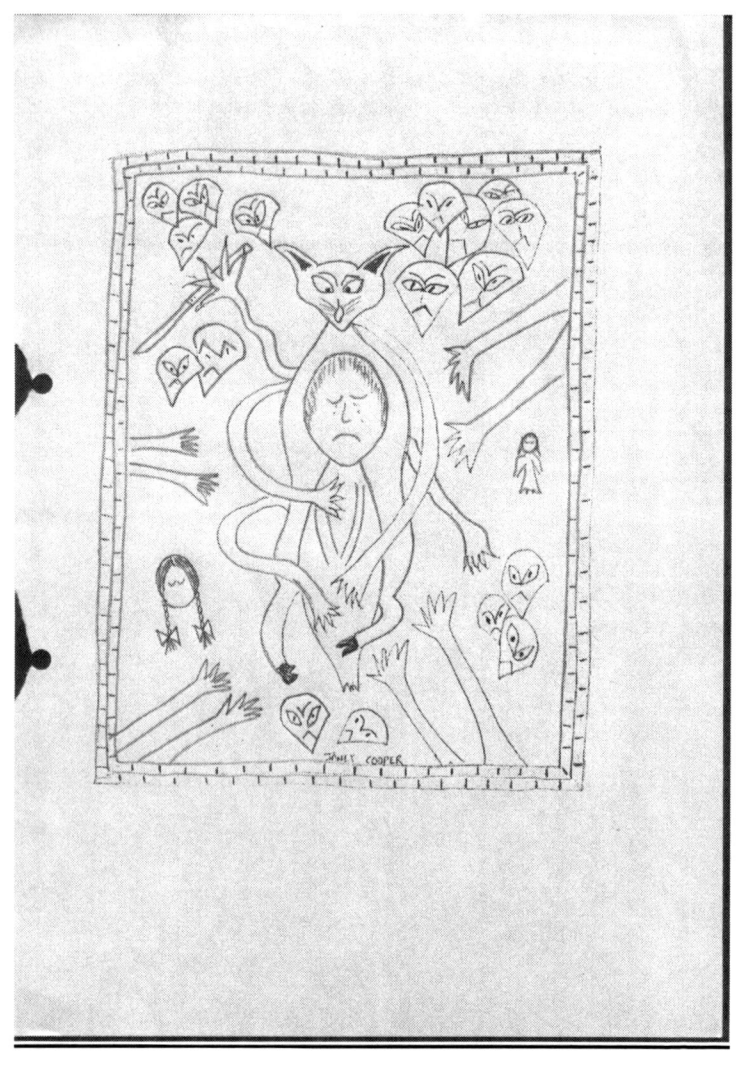

THE HUDDLE

CHAPTER SIX   FOOD FOR THE HUDDLE

Food for The Huddle? Yep. This was certainly my planned title for this next chapter. Little did I realise that they would be feeding upon me voraciously when I had wanted to begin typing. So the typing was delayed, and not until today have I been bothered to make the enormous effort to plug in my typewriter and summon up the energy required to type. Even now I feel, what is the point? What is the point of typing anything? What is the point of anything? Anything, anything at all that requires my lungs to continue breathing and my heart to beat is a waste of time. Concrete head. I am down down, deep in a pit.

Not as low as yesterday or the day before or the day before that. But low, low down. Depression. A banquet for The Huddle, and how they love me when I am like this! I am the most delicious of food for them whilst in this sorry, pathetic state, and they pick on me and consume me with much slurping, slobbering and enjoyment. Angel says to type how I feel. Rachel tells me to get lost. The Huddle tell me to kill myself because I'm already dead anyway! It might be possible today to write down how I feel. Not too sure though. Concentration isn't brilliant. Each sentence takes ages to write if it is to make any sense.

I could pick any one member of The Huddle and say, "He teareth me in his wrath, who hateth me: he gnasheth upon me with his teeth: mine enemy sharpeneth his eyes upon me. ….." The Huddle have "gathered themselves together against me. God hath delivered me to the ungodly, and turned me over into the hands of the wicked." "My face is foul with weeping, and on my eyelids is the shadow of death." My breath is corrupt, my days are extinct, the graves are ready for me." "I have made my bed in darkness." "And where is now my hope? As for my hope, who shall see it? They shall go down to the bars of the pit, where our rest together is in the dust." (From Job)

Rachel's depression has seeped malignantly from her cell and poured itself into my mind. I am filled with darkness and have no hope because there is no hope. The hours are gloomy years that offer not a glimmer of relief. Ever! My body is slow and unwilling to move. I do not want to do anything. I do not want to do this typing. My heart is broken and cannot be mended. I pine for the light I cannot have.   Unshed tears build up inside my head and it shall surely explode. Yesterday I kept bursting into tears. Today I cannot cry. But pressure in my head. Awful, bad pressure. Crushing. Unrelenting. Tormenting. I am in agony.

I am sat at my desk and as I type I have on my headphones. Listening to J.S.Bach. Huddle bad. Too bad. Type away! Clack, clack, clack. Listen to the music. Listen to that. Listen to that; drown them out, out, out, voices, voices, voices, voices…….

I am not alone. Rachel is crying bitterly. I am indescribably lonely, watching fingers move over keys but not feeling as if they belong to me. They are separate. Not me. I am a thing trapped inside a living body I do not want. I wish it was as dead and rotting as I am. Why does it not give up?

If I was truly loved, then the people who say they love me would let me go. Please, all of you let

THE HUDDLE

me go! Hate me, loathe me, detest me, do anything but love me, for then I could go. My pain is unbearable. Do you understand? Nothing is real any more. Only this dark agony. Reality, whatever reality is, no longer exists. The world goes on like some evil game that is nothing but a delusion. I would like to melt into someone, be absorbed by them, be eaten up, sucked in and destroyed so that I no longer exist. Be surrounded by tight arms and disappear forever. Take over for me. I cannot go on. I *need* to cease to exist. Take me away. Away from everything. Away. Please!

I have nothing. Even my children are no longer real to me. How *can* they be mine? They are distant. Separate. Me in a glass bubble looking out. In pain. In too much pain. It is so wrong for me to agree to exist much longer in this state. Screaming, rotting, stark staring agony. Keep typing, clack, clack, voices, voices, keep listening to the music, music, keep on listening, voices, voices, voices, Huddle, Huddle, must not go on with this…

Too many. Too long. Cannot bear for much longer. Worms will come. Peeking at me now. Slimy heads. Pink. Feel sick, don't care, nothing matters, voices, voices…

If I had a physical agony then I would look forward to my next analgesic dose. Would that at least give some relief, if only for a few hours? But my pain is mental and so I have nothing to look forward to; no promise of relief. Ever. Nothing. No relief, no hope, voices, voices, darkness, this terrible pressure inside my head building up and up and up and voices and too dark and too heavy…

The thought that I might still be alive one hour from now is a bad one; unbearable to me, I cannot bear to stay alive for another hour! I want a rest. I want *the* rest! Long, long rest.

Will I please be shot? Somebody shoot me, shoot me, shoot me, please, and voices go on and laugh and me want to scream now and **SMASH** our useless head against the nearest, hardest, thickest brick wall. Smash foul brains out of this obscene existence. A dog would be put out of its misery. Why not me? Am I not worth killing?? Is it not worth relieving my torment??? Obviously not...

Voices, voices, voices, voices, voices...................

I am left. Abandoned. Discarded. Everybody conspires against me. They all want me like this. They do not care. They do not do anything about it. They smile and live lives. They do not really love me. They will not let me go. There is no usefulness, no value and no point in being this way. It is not right.

Lord, if you love me then take The Huddle from me! I am whining to you like a spoilt child!! Better still, just take *me*! Please!!! All the day long they pick at me. They ridicule me and scorn me. I am their meat day and night. How long *will* You look on and do nothing??

God? See me when I have lain down on the ground and they have covered me like flies, consuming me, permeating my rotting carcass with squirming maggots that eat my decaying flesh. For Christ's sake, can't you smell the stench of this soul

THE HUDDLE

destroying, decomposing depression? Feel my soggy, stinking flesh! Hear them that mock my deadly state. How long must I die for? How long must I be dead for? Feel my pain as only You can, and take pity on my wretched state.

I do not live. I do not love. I do not want my existence as it is. Why doesn't God take my unshed tears, purify them in heaven and wash me with them so that I will be whiter than snow? Why doesn't He stop my ears so that I cannot hear the voices? Why isn't Jesus a sweet smell to me? What have I done that I am like this? Heavy, awful, too hopeless, there is no comfort, none give me comfort, all are far off and separate and never can reach me or touch me.

Each person within me is tormented. Depression. Torture. Satan torments us. Our past torments us. Me and them are punished. Punished for being a me and an us. We are loathed and hated. The world is against us. Does not want us. We do not want it. Cannot type much more.

Listen to the music, listen to it, keep listening to it. I don't know what I am going to do. I do not want to be alive an hour from now. I shall not be able to bear that. No point, no point in anything, no point, no point, voices, voices, too dark now and lots of tablets in the cupboard.

Angel says, "Please don't Janet, please don't!" but I want, I want, I want... I want a pair of gold shoes but I cannot have them. I would spoil them. No point.

It is now Thursday. Today is better than yesterday. Today I will not kill me. Yesterday I was not sure that I wouldn't do that evil thing. My evil comforter is gone and I have to keep being reminded of that. "He is gone!" Says Angel. How gently she reminds me, knowing that his loss is so mourned by me at times. I think Angel is a copy of Dr. Kapp's voice. She says the sort of stuff Dr. Kapp would say, so is this my mind's way of psychotherapying the gaps between my psychiatrist's visits?

The Huddle continue to feed upon this foul depression with great relish. I feel unable and unwilling to help myself. Neither do I want to be helped. There's no point, and yet I willingly sit and type today. I have also tried to read, having come across a little book that belongs to Frank. It's a tiny book, only having fifteen pages, and is called 'Unspoken Prayer'. Some of the lines it contains 'spoke' to me. Listen to this. (That is if you're still reading and in spite of your boredom are determined to carry on reading!)

"Are we so overwhelmed that we cannot even groan or sigh? So low that we cannot give vent to even a tear or a look? So utterly cold, inert and hopeless that the soul feels it is prayerless? Yet, surely there must be a desire after God..." Perhaps today I can reply with some words from the prophet Isaiah. "With my soul have I desired thee (God) in the night." Maybe when I slept and was not aware of me, then something or someone about me cried out to God for help???
Who knows?

At least today I have cried and found it less of an effort to move my body. The darkness is not such impenetrable gloom and yet the chink of light

THE HUDDLE

frightens me. What if I like it and it does not last? Like the time before, and the time before that, and the time even before the time before that…….

There have been chinks of light, but they do not last. There is no greater misery than to remember a time of joy and light when you are again shrouded in darkness and another dark night of the soul presses upon you. That is a worse agony; better never to have seen the light at all! Safer the devil you know, lest your last state be worse than your first.

So yes. I have a desire towards God. I recognise that today and I pine for Him. Groaning, pining and longing that does not feel heard, answered or satisfied. The Huddle, predictably, strive against this desire of mine and so I'm a battle ground once more and with the scars to prove it. I am wounded and in agony. I am also in a state of self pity, of giving up, of not coping too well, of not even wanting to cope, and of wanting to be taken away from all this.

I want a pair of gold shoes; symbolic of a prettier walk through life. "…feet shod with the preparation of the Gospel of peace." (Ephesians 6:15) Peace. Peace means no Huddle. No rotting depression. No sharing of my body or my mind in any way. Knowing I am forgiven and acceptable to God. Peace! I want my gold shoes! I have seen them, the prettiest gold shoes ever! They almost mock me from the shop window because they know I cannot have them. But really, it is The Huddle that mock me. Not the beautiful shoes.

The muddle that's The Huddle!! They are always at me. Watching me. Talking *to* me and about me.

Commenting about what I do and what I don't do. "Lazy f**king bitch!" And worse. So much worse. You know. You remember what I've typed previously. Do you? Or have you already forgotten most of it? I am not able to forget them.

They constantly remind me of how evil, blasphemous and obscene they are; evil satanic minions grown so big and powerful and overwhelming to me. Voices, voices, a huddle of voices, demonic prattlers, enemies of my soul, voices, voices, on and on and on and on and on and on and on and on and on and on and on and on and on and on and on and on and on and on and on…… fed up with me typing that? Yes. I'm fed up of it too. Maybe you didn't bother to read every 'and' and every 'on'. That's your choice, and you're free to make it. You can quickly pass over the bits you find boring. I can't do that! The Huddle are incredibly boring, on and on, but I cannot choose to get away from them. They will not leave me alone and are wearing me down. I feel worn out and exhausted from the constant battle. I want a rest but there is no rest. I can't put them down or abandon them – you could do either with this book – even chuck it in the bin! You, dear reader, are in control of how much of The Huddle you want to put up with. I envy you….

The Huddle hates me and calls me names. "Sticks and stones may break my bones but names will never hurt me." Huh! That must be one of the most untrue sayings of all time! Please!!! Give me the broken bones instead! At least there's a good chance they will heal – but my mind? The names are killing me. They are hurting me. The Huddle

THE HUDDLE

torment me night and day and I am in agony. Foul enemies!

Now I am thinking of the last verse of one of my favourite hymns.

"The soul that on Jesus has leaned for repose,
I will not, I will not desert to its foes.
That soul, though all hell should endeavour to shake,
I'll never, no never, no never forsake!"

But…   but Lord? You *have* forsaken me and left me to The Huddle!!

WHY AM I LIKE THIS?????????????

"S**t on her! Another f**king po bloody em! What she……."

Oh! How the privileged soul rejoices!
The one that does not hear the voices,
Spitting, spagging,
Swearing, nagging,
Whisper, hate her,
Shout to kill her,
Vitriolic, angry, darkly
Glaring at you
Glaring back.

So up I get from cosy bed
To flee the torments of my head
But I can not. The voices follow me
And say I'll rot
In hell.

Janet Cooper

And so I rot.
They laugh and smirk and jeer,
"Don't look behind you!
Satan's near!"

A demon tumbles from the ceiling,
I'm terrified, my head is reeling.
In front of me an evil Janny,
Hands bleeding, calling "Mammy! Mammy!"
And into me she comes.

And all the while imprisoned Rachel
Claws away my brain,
We feel we'll go insane.
The cell wherein she rants and raves
Is in my head. A row of graves
Awaits all voices in this head.
That's relief!
Be dead,
Be dead.

I am not comforted tonight.
I'm hand in hand with fear
And he's so near, so very near,
And so again, again, again
There is no comforter.
There is no cuddle, is no hug
To ease the voices in my head.
O please! Please God or Satan or whoever,
Please be kind and strike me dead!

I take a little pill instead,
Chemical relief for poorly head.
It doesn't always work.

THE HUDDLE

And then go back to bed and cry a silent tear
Whilst listening to a crowd.
I'm lonely! O, so lonely in this crowded mind.
Please let me go to sleep and leave behind…..
Myself.

I wrote that in the middle of yet another sleepless night, so I must be feeling better or else I would not write anything! It is now the weekend. This book seems to be turning into some sort of 'Diary of a Depression!" So what. Does not matter. I'm writing about how life is for me with The Huddle, so it's still relevant. But am I even sure any longer about why I'm bothering to write all this in the first place? Oh yes, of course I am. It's catharsis; one of my coping mechanisms, but it didn't stop me getting depressed and it didn't stop the voices getting worse, did it! A coping method can only be a coping method as long as I am coping!! Make sense? Probably not. Anyway, back to the subject of this chapter.

As the previous boringly miserable pages lucidly point out, depression is one of the things about me/us that The Huddle feeds on hungrily. Even bulimically! Gorging themselves and verbally vomiting into my mind. My lowered mood makes them stronger, louder and more tormenting. I am weakened by mental pain and find that I do not resist them or tune out of them so easily. The big question is, do I get depressed because the voices become worse, or do the voices become worse *because* I am depressed? It's like the age old enquiry over which comes first, the chicken or the egg!

Personally, I believe the chicken came first! I also believe that a lot of my depressive episodes are due to the fact that I get fed up with The Huddle to the point where I would do anything just to have a rest from them. I get sick of it all, sick of them, sick of having to cope, sick of the constant effort to be okay, and sick of myself. (Yeh, I know, I've probably told you this loads of times so far. Remember! Catharsis!! Remember! However bored you may be reading this – how much more 'bored' am I?) So I stop caring what happens to me, I stop making so much effort to fight back, and I start to give up and sink into them and then wallow in the pain and misery and self pity of it all. I hate myself, I hate them, I hate the way I am and my continued existence seems of no value. There really is no point in me living and no usefulness to be gained from spending another second in the company of The Huddle! And if I'm repeating myself yet again, then GOOD!!

Therefore I become depressed. The Huddle know I am depressed and that my defences are down, hence they become worse. They seize their chance to torment me all the more whilst I have not the physical or mental energy to tune out of them. So they feed on me, holistically, mind, body and soul. They feed on the *real* me.

The Huddle also feed and gain strength from specific things about me, like my anger, which I have already mentioned at length, and my unforgiveness. Now that's a big issue with me and one that causes a lot of misery. The Bible tells me that unless I forgive others, then God will not forgive me, and for my own peace of mind I need to

THE HUDDLE

forgive and be forgiven for so many things. I do not feel that I have this forgiveness and therefore I see myself as unacceptable to God. I am not 'right' with Him because I do not forgive others. But again I would ask, how do you forgive a rapist? How? Also, if that rapist has not asked God to forgive him, then how can God expect me to forgive somebody that God Himself has not forgiven? Am I higher than God? I don't think so. And if God forgives absolutely anything, can't He forgive my unforgiveness????? (Did you read that last sentence Reverend H.? Are you reading this?? If so, then you shouldn't be! For you told me this sort of writing was not glorifying to God – remember how you made me burn some of my writing in your living-room fire? Therefore if it's 'sin' for me to write, then it is surely greater 'sin' for a 'minister of God' to read – especially if you've got this far. SO THERE!!!!!!!)

Can't carry on now. They are telling me to shut up and soon there will be worms like the ones that oozed out of the pages of a book last night, and then we went to bed and dreamed of large black beetles crawling out of the holes of my little oil burner. I woke up and tried to brush the beetles off my pillow. Frank reassured me, through a haze of sleep, that I was alright, so I snuggled down, risking them crawling all over my face. I could not feel them but I knew that they were there. Shall I ever be able to continue with the subject of this chapter?
"F**king well NO! Dull bitch, fat witch, she's not SUPPOSED to be writing about US!!! … we F**king

get her … ugly cow soon stop that frigging typing … go rip the s*dding stuff up …"

I am not yet undepressed enough to sit and concentrate and type for any length of time, but then what's the use of anything I do anyway?

I am blank. I am scared. I have a bad head. Voices. Pressure. Very black ahead and all around. I can't do anything. I have been very depressed and I have cried and she has cried and there is no point in me going on. I must be alive because my body moves. Nevertheless it is not how I feel or how I want to be. There is no life inside my head! I live only to function for the benefit (!!???????????????!!) of Frank and two children. It feels like there is no *real* me. Just a head. A full head that aches a lot. I am, I see, I feel nothing pretty. No prettiness or colours. Pressure. Terrible pressure. I don't know what to do. I mustn't type any more. Perhaps they have won…..

Now it is days later. It is Monday. Aumonier wrote;

I will seek beauty all my days.
Within the dark chaos of a troubled world I will
Seek and find some beauteous thing.
From eyes grown dim with weeping shall shine a light
To guide me, and in sorrows hour
I shall behold a great High courage.
I shall find the wonder of an infinite Patience
And a quiet Faith in coming Joy and Peace.
And love will I seek in the midst of discord, and
Find swift eager hands outstretched in welcome.

THE HUDDLE

I will seek beauty all my days, and in my quest
I shall not be dismayed.
I SHALL FIND GOD!

That is so very lovely and does not require me to pass any other comment. I shall not spoil the beautiful words by typing what The Huddle are now saying. Now it is time to put on my headphones and read again those amazing words.

Today is a better day. "Let me be delivered from them that hate me, and out of the deep waters." (Psalm 69:14)

I SHALL FIND GOD! (Many thanks, Aumonier, whoever you were!)

I also saw our psychiatrist today. That should have been 'my' psychiatrist seeing as I am writing this account as me. But no matter, I'm not going to edit it out, as that's how 'life' is! I am an us. Damn it!!

Dr. Kapp and I spoke about Christmas, which is now only a matter of weeks away. I never plan to be alive at Christmas time, but I've obviously been a lousy, cowardly planner and now that I have lost my evil comforter all that thinking *has* to change. This year *has* to be different and better. What's the alternative? But *how?*

I asked Dr. Kapp, "Do you *enjoy* Christmas?" and her face lit up.

"Yes!" she responded, immediately, "I love Christmas!"

What??? I was surprisingly delighted by her answer! No help would she have been to me if she'd been one of the many people for whom this time of year is nothing but a chore, or perhaps even a time of great unhappiness. Dr. Kapp managed to kindle within me a little joy and excitement towards the coming yuletide and I am now approaching the season with a little more hope. I am daring to hope! She has so encouraged me that I am determined that this Christmas will not be another opportunity for misery and scrooge-ish attitudes. I shall attempt the proverbial 'snap out of it' and if that doesn't work than I shall win an Oscar for my acting! My children deserve my effort, even if I don't. This year *will* be different. But...

Where the Huddle delighted and fed upon my misery, they will hate and attempt to spoil my positive efforts, crushing out all joy. So help me God. I cannot escape them.

Okay. Back to the chapter topic! Where I had hoped to categorise the things about me on which the Huddle feed, I now realise that that would be inappropriate and take forever. Because there isn't actually much about me that they *don't* feed on! If I am angry, they will feed upon my anger, making it worse, and then accusing me of it. If I am *not* angry they will invade any measure of peace I have managed to attain and deliberately *make* me angry. And then accuse me of it! Either way they get a good meal. They even feed upon the 'normal' things about me; things that I cannot avoid. Like, I have to eat, wash and go to the toilet.

"Don't eat, fat bitch, dirty bitch, s**tting bitch..."

THE HUDDLE

Like, I have one head, two arms and two legs.

"Two legged f**king freak!"

My lungs breathe and my heart beats.

"Evil, beating frigging pump rump, go stop it, go stop it...."

Me in totality is food for The Huddle! They pick at me, chew away on me, gaining strength and sustenance from all my weaknesses, inadequacies and sin. They have spoiled anything that might have been strong and good about me and turned those attributes into a veritable feast to sustain them in their miserable and pathetic existence.

I am food for them! In order to be Huddle free it would appear that I would need to be perfect and sinless, but even that might not get rid of them for they would goad me into sin, tempt me and taunt me. And besides which, it is humanly impossible for me to be perfect and sinless "for all have sinned and fall short of the glory of God".

The Bible promises that out of weakness shall come strength, but in my case, not strength for me but strength for The Huddle. I feel I am in a no win situation with them holding all the aces. I cannot win and there is no way out but one, and that I cannot take.

Food for the Huddle? ***I AM THEIR FOOD, DAMN IT!!!!!!!!!!*** I am their constant supply. Everything about me sustains them and keeps them going. Could they exist without me for food? Interesting question! Do I need to exist in order for them to exist? Without me, would they seek out some other unfortunate victim, or would they, also, shrivel up and die some final death?

Janet Cooper

I'm probably getting boring by keeping on now, but ... it is sickening! The way the Huddle are always feeding on me. Constantly sucking, biting, chewing and picking. They binge on my depressions, my self pity, my hopelessness, my anger, my unforgiveness, my bitterness, my hatred, my fear. If I got rid of all these bad bits, would they torment me less because there was less to feed on? The misery, guilt and shame I feel over my past provides a positive banquet for them, liberally flavoured with nightmares and flashbacks, my tears their condiments as they stuff them selves to overflowing, becoming big and gross and huge and heavy. Gluttons of my soul, they leave their teeth marks upon me and my mind drips their foul saliva. I am a bulimic binge that swells them to gigantic, uncomfortable proportions when they will vomit their filth into my ears, polluting me with their overindulgence in obscenity, blasphemy and cruelty. They spill out and regurgitate their vile waste, flooding me with their sickening and constant tirade. They are never empty. Sometimes I want to heave and retch and vomit them right out of me, getting rid of their badness. They have voracious appetites, not caring that I decay and rot as they will still eat. They are evil. They are pathetic, boring and persistent. Why? WHY?? **WHY???**

Something has just occurred to me. By hating me, The Huddle also hate the food that they feed upon. What a thought! Therefore, is it possible to make their food even more obnoxious to them by dealing positively with my anger, unforgiveness etc.? By more diligently seeking after God, will I

THE HUDDLE

become so unpalatable to them that they will go? But yet I *do* seek after God! This reasoning would imply that I make no effort whatsoever, which surely can't be true? I can't be any more sorry for what I've done that's wrong. The only reason I don't seek more diligently after God is *because* of The Huddle! And I would ask again – anyone out there! – How can I forgive the man who raped me? I wish I wanted to forgive him, but I can't even get as far as that at the moment. So according to Rev.H.'s God, I remain unforgiven myself and not right with God. Hence The Huddle. Harsh theology! As one of his congregation once whispered to me, "He's more Calvinistic than Calvin!" It was not meant as a compliment!!

Something else has just occurred to me. Do The Huddle know unimaginable misery by being forced to live with me and eat food which they hate? To be so constantly hungry that they have to swallow food that is abhorrent to them must be torment, surely! When you stop to think about it, what a terrible existence The Huddle have! Their lives are taken up with torment and rotten food! How dreadful! Yet I cannot feel an ounce of pity for them. What have *they* done to be in such a pathetic and miserable situation?

I used to think that if I could give The Huddle to someone then I would. Now I am not so sure. Well, maybe I would give them to certain people from my past that have hurt me so dreadfully.

"Cruel f**king bitch … she lousy Christian … not love, cruel bitch, cruel bitch, cruel bitch…"

Frank would take them from me if he could. That is love. But if he had them just for one day, would he change his mind?

If they are feeding off me then they are not feeding off and tormenting anybody else. Can this be a more useful way to look at my situation? Dive into altruism! Do the world a favour and keep your damn voices to yourself. Become a martyr to The Huddle! Oh, I don't know!!!! My concentration is going a bit now. Angel says to finish this chapter. Okay then.

THE END OF THIS BORING CHAPTER

This chapter is not how I'd planned to write it. I fear it is boring, repetitive and makes little sense, but I don't want to destroy it because that's exactly what The Huddle are telling me to do. I don't feel as if I've explained myself very well or written anything that was worth writing other than for purpose of catharsis. (So therefore it's been worth writing!!!) Doesn't really matter. This is *my* book. My therapy. It can be this way…….

The Huddle are now back in my desk lamp. I am so sick of them. I have turned off the lamp and turned the bulb away from me and they have laughed at my efforts to repel them. Futile efforts!

But remember this, wretched voices,
> I shall not be dismayed,
> I SHALL FIND GOD!!!!!

THE HUDDLE

There is no life, no living, inside my head. Only the voices and the others. That is existence. Not life. I forced me to draw sky and grass in colour. But the colour is not real or pretty for me. I don't know what will happen to me.

CHAPTER SEVEN   MY PSYCHIATRIST AND OTHER COPING STRATEGIES.

Strategy. The art or science of the planning and conduct of a war.
Stratagem. A plan or trick, especially to deceive an enemy.

These are appropriate words with which to describe my methods of coping with The Huddle. They *are* my enemy, and every day I have to be alert, and planning to stay one step ahead of them if I am to continue to function at a reasonable level. I am indeed conducting a war!

I have mentioned some of my coping mechanisms in previous chapters but would like to discuss them in greater detail. Although there are specific things I spend time doing every day in order to tune out of these wretched voices, almost anything can be turned into a coping mechanism if I am desperate enough. Even some simple tasks such as cleaning my teeth! It involves having to super concentrate on everything I am doing, throwing my whole mind into whatever activity, and that can really help to keep The Huddle in the background. Nevertheless, it takes constant effort to do this, it's exhausting, and I can never fully relax. Take brushing my teeth as an example…

Toothpaste, what colour? White. Smell it, smells minty, so onto toothbrush, pink toothbrush, squeeze the paste out. In a line. Brush top teeth and think about taste. Count the brushstrokes, turn the tap on and listen to the water, listen, listen,

THE HUDDLE

brush teeth, think about the taste and keep listening to the water, up and down, up and down, across, across, bottom teeth now, brush hard, hear the brush scrubbing my teeth, frothy minty toothpaste now, listen to the water, watch the water, nice taste..... Et cetera.

To force myself to become over engrossed in any task *is* helpful, but it is also extremely boring. For example, there is a limit to how interesting cleaning teeth can be! It also means I have a constant struggle to keep my mind so busy that it is too otherwise occupied to take any notice of The Huddle. It is certainly very tiring, but rather that than 'bad Huddle'. I nearly always have a headache, which I suppose is hardly surprising.

Other ways of coping can be more time consuming. They include listening to music with headphones on, exercise, the use of a mantra, writing, playing the piano and reading, although the reading depends on how my concentration is at any time. I love to read, so it is a misery to me when I can't!! Imagine trying to concentrate on a book when a crowd of people are yelling at you. Oh yes, I almost forgot, writing this book is also another big coping method. I relish the constant clack, clack, clack of the typewriter, but like any other method of coping, The Huddle can be saboteurs, turning my efforts into food.

They are, for example, fighting against the writing of this book because I find it therapeutic to discuss them with an imaginary reader, and they hate that! Often, now, it is a battle to keep the clacking going! Will I finish a few pages before they make it too much of a misery for me and the worms appear to scare me off? Why don't I, at their kind suggestion, abandon the idea of writing this book now that it is becoming a struggle for me? Well, why should I give it up? Why should I give in to them? To do so would simply make matters worse as they will have gained a useful victory and I shall have failed. Thus more food for them!! No way am I going to let that happen! It is better to grit my teeth and fight on.

Angel says that the fight I am in is a good one. I don't know whether I believe *that*! We are now thinking of that hymn,
"Fight the good fight with all thy might,
Christ is thy strength and Christ thy right."

Why then does Christ not take on this battle for me? I thought His death on the cross had brought victory. For whom? I am still fighting.

I am self pitying. Again.

My best loved coping method is my psychiatrist. It is unfair of me to refer to her as a coping method because she is so much more. She is an intelligent, loving and wonderful human being who gives me so much more than any of my other strategies for getting through the days. My music centre does not love me, smile at me, or give me hugs. Neither can I have so precious a relationship with my Libby Roberts aerobic tape! I am glad I have my piano, but I don't exactly care about it as I care about my psychiatrist. Many times I'd love to give her a quick kick on the shin, many times I exhort her to stop hurrying, because she'll wear herself out! We have a very specific and unique relationship.

Unlike my other coping mechanisms I cannot employ Dr. Kapp at will. I have to wait for her to arrive and be totally accepting as to how often she is willing and able to see us. At the moment I see her once every two or three weeks and this would seem perfectly adequate. I no longer need our intense weekly sessions. Prior to her arrival I'll have a quick tidy round, make sure I'm clean and neat (so she'll know I'm okay, functioning adequately, taking care over my appearance etc. etc.) and think through all The Huddle muck and emotional garbage I am desperate to offload on her. Dr. Kapp does, however, leave my mind usefully scattered with psychological nuggets which I can chew away at between her visits (is that Angel's role? Is Angel a Dr. Kapp of my psyche??).

I'm all ready to talk, talk, talk when Dr. Kapp arrives, but I inevitably fall silent as soon as we both sit opposite each other and the 'hellos' are over.

"Shut your mouth! F**king mouthy bitch! She talk but no-one interested in sick bitch witch bitch………"

Prolific on paper, I am not a good talker and so I sit quietly and wait for her to nudge me into opening my mouth. Then we talk and talk. It is so very relieving to be able to share how I am with somebody else and for an hour every few weeks my malady is no longer a closely guarded secret; it's out in the open and I can say whatever I want to say. For me anyway, this time together is a very precious privilege.

Sometimes, too, we sit a while with neither of us saying a word. This can be very good as well. How can I describe that? Like a wordless sharing of how

I am; a depth of understanding that requires no verbal expression. Maybe prayer? I don't know.

As you can no doubt imagine, The Huddle do not like Dr. Kapp (are there any people they *do* like?). In fact they hate her. Surprise, surprise! They hate the fact that she knows all about them and supports me in my efforts to cope with their constant abuse. They are especially livid because Dr. Kapp would like to see me free of them and all the restrictions they impose on my life. So, what do they do about this? They attempt to sabotage my therapeutic relationship with her, at times achieving a measure of success. The Huddle tell me that she secretly hates me and doesn't care two hoots what happens to me. According to them, Dr. Kapp wishes she didn't have to come and sit with me, as I'm nothing but an extra chore and burden tagged on to her already overloaded NHS work. It is so easy for me to believe all this, but I've also thought of Dr. Kapp more as 'God sent' rather than 'NHS sent', so therefore, in obedience to God, she could not refuse to see me! (Still doesn't mean that I wouldn't be an unwanted chore! I must be a bit like cleaning the loo – you wish you didn't have to do it, but you do it because you have to, or else live with unpleasant consequences.) I still reckon that of her own choosing, Dr. Kapp would prefer not to have met me. Simply because I am me, us, and not worth bothering with.

The Huddle do not help when it comes to the matter of my rock bottom self esteem. Neither does Rachel, who will frequently and smugly announce that "Dr. Kapp likes me better than she likes you! So there!" Am I jealous? You bet! Of course I am! I

THE HUDDLE

can be extremely childish at times. Rachel has certain qualities I do not possess. When not depressed she can be endearingly outspoken and animated, and to hear her play the piano, you would not believe she uses the same fingers I use!

The Huddle love to tell me things about Dr. Kapp that I know cannot possibly be true, yet nonetheless can be extremely distressing both to me and to Rachel. They show her to me in my dreams in a way meant to cause horror, disgust, dislike, and a desire never to see her again. They also torment me by saying that I am bad for her, knowing me will cause her great harm, and I am a jinx and a misery to spend time with. It is all very cruel. Dr. Kapp is not at all how they draw her in my mind and I am always relieved when she turns up looking and acting like herself, even if I am a little wary of her for the first few minutes!

The Huddle also tell me things about her that just might *be* true! I don't know. Like she lives at 'The Munster's', has size seven feet and her favourite biscuits are Ginger Nuts! Yes. I can see a funny side to this sort of thing, much to The Huddle's frustration. Funny, yes, but think about it a little more just for a minute or two, because The Huddle don't tell me anything with the intention of causing me some amusement at their expense, do they!

The Munster's!! It's a dirty, dingy, creepy, haunted house inhabited by a bunch of peculiars! Living there, Dr. Kapp would be dressed in sinister black and be a lover of tombs, death and the occult. She would delight in all things abnormal. (Perhaps psychiatrists do??) All this is not necessarily a funny picture to somebody who has dabbled in the occult!

Why size seven feet, I hear you ask. Easy! Seven is God's number, and one degree up on the Devil's 666. One moment Dr. Kapp is Dr. Horrible, next moment The Huddle are sarcastically portraying her as some exceptional goody goody.

"Holy f**king bitch sent by holy f**king God is here... shod with the f**king preparation of the f**king Gospel of f**king peace....Size seven holy f**king shod feet on..."

It's not funny. Then why Ginger Nut biscuits? I used to be a coppery, gingery colour years ago before a few grey strands appeared and I began a love affair with harmony hair colour. I am also a nut!

"She likes you, she likes her, gonna swallow her whole! What she gonna do to ginger Nut? F**king barmy biscuit, Ginger Nut, she loves f**king Ginger Nuts ... know what we mean, sad cow?"

Their miserable obscenity is not the least bit funny when heard in these sorts of contexts.

I was amazed at how deeply hurt and upset Rachel was to hear that Dr. Kapp lives at 'The Munster's'. I wonder did she ever watch the television series with me, though possibly not, as she can see not one funny side to all this. Unfortunately, and so childishly, I wound her up with silly tales of our psychiatrist brewing spells in a cobweb infested kitchen, circle dancing in the garden with a bunch of weirdoes (could have been her colleagues?) and tucking into an extra rare steak with Herman Munster while her little dogs sat on the coffee table and howled! At times I forget

THE HUDDLE

that Rachel is a very hurt and damaged seventeen year old and could not cope with this sort of cruel teasing. She was frightened that Dr. Kapp's spells were to get rid of her and the circle dancing and eating of 'raw' meat equated to membership of a coven. I should not have done it to Rachel, I know that now, but part of me still finds it funny. At least I'm honest!! The thing is, The Huddle had set out to further distress me but I had managed to turn at least some of it into a source of amusement, however wrong and inappropriate.

Dreams about Dr. Kapp can be incredibly sad and painful. The worst ones are repetitive still. I don't know whether to write about some of them as she will possibly read this, but I am brave today and she isn't coming for another week and that is a long, long time away.

In one dream, she is kneeling on the floor and crying bitterly. Jesus is stood away in the distance and behind Him are two shadows. I know that one is her husband and the other is a small child. They are both in heaven. I am watching and waiting for Jesus to comfort Dr. Kapp, for I know that He will, but I am not allowed to see this and get very upset. So I go to put my arms out to her, but The Huddle push me away.

Another dream shows her in a room that is large and cold. There is an angel on one wall and a pretty chandelier hangs from the ceiling and twinkles. Dr. Kapp sits there alone while the angel watches her before the two of them make their way to Dr. Kapp's car. (I can see this dream as wanting my psychiatrist looked after because she's useful to me!!)

Yet another dream shows me in the living-room of Dr. Kapp's cottage in North Yorkshire. When I first started having this dream I was always very pregnant in it and about to give birth. Now I am sometimes pregnant, and sometimes not, but always I know that I am about to give birth to something and make the most terrible mess. I don't know how to clean this mess up and I am on the way to the public phone to tell Dr. Kapp about it. Positive that she will be extremely angry with me, I am frantic and in a panic, crying as I dial her number. Other dreams horribly glorify The Huddle and I don't want to record them.

Dr. Kapp also helps me to cope by taking the time to talk to the other personalities. Rachel and Liz have always called her Elinor, whereas it took me a very long time to do this. Katy calls her Dr. Kapp, and little Janny refers to her as either Ellie or Mrs Ellie. I know all this because Rachel has told me, knowing more about the others than I do. Apparently Janny talks to her 'rab rab' about Dr. Ellie. "You gotta be a *very* good rab rab, or I tell Dr. Ellie!"

I don't know *how* Dr. Kapp talks to Liz, Katy or Janny but I do know that when she wants to talk to Rachel then she will simply call her by name. When she does so, she always closes her eyes as if she's concentrating and this makes me feel ridiculously cut off and excluded. Not wanted. Childish I know, but that's how I feel. I do not like the transition from me to Rachel and will try to fight against it happening. At least I have come to feel relatively safe with Dr. Kapp and have asked her to please make absolutely sure it is 'me' when she leaves

THE HUDDLE

otherwise I feel confused and abandoned without so much as a goodbye.

Becoming absent is a weird feeling. Sometimes it will happen suddenly, even without Dr. Kapp expecting it, but more often I will experience a feeling of confusion, of Rachel struggling to speak out of my mouth, and then there is nothing. It's like being under an anaesthetic when time simply disappears and you have no idea of what is going on. Only very rarely have I known what Rachel has spoken about. I never know what Liz, Katy or Janny say. I am absent. I lose time.

It can be very disturbing and distressing not knowing what your body has done or said. I am now hearing Rachel in my right ear. She is reading what I type with great interest.

"I am not your bloody *body*! I'm **ME**!!"

Rachel is thankfully far less depressed this week and has been playing the piano, making beds, wiping the dishes, and wanting to know what's going on again. I suppose this is a good thing. Change that! This *is* a good thing!

During some sessions when Dr. Kapp has spoken to one of them I have 'come back' to find that everything on the coffee table has been swept onto the carpet. On one occasion a saucer was smashed. Always when Dr. Kapp has spoken to Rachel I will find myself no longer sitting on my chair but crouched on the settee next to my doctor. My eyes might be puffy with crying and there will usually be a pile of soggy tissues on the arm of the settee. I will feel as if I have suddenly emerged from a dark cinema into the daylight! Everything will appear unreal and far away, Dr. Kapp will be sat there smiling (because it isn't happening to her!) and I will snatch a quick glance at the clock to see how much time has passed.

I will nearly always ask, "What have I done?" or "Who have you spoken to?" and I will be given only a brief outline as most of what the others say I do not want to know about. In this respect I can see that they are also a coping mechanism for me; a self defence of the psyche, each having their own memories, their own autobiographies. If I had to carry all their fears and memories as well as my own, than I should be mad.

I am an us in order that they each may preserve the whole, and it makes a lot of sense for it to be this way. I would not survive as an 'I'. The others have gone through parts of the life this body has experienced so that the whole has not collapsed under too great an emotional trauma. Yes, it does make sense to me and how I wish I was better at describing what I mean! It is most certainly *not* a disorder! It is extremely *ordered*! However, I have to concede that it isn't perceived as normality when you are not in control of your body at all times. Think about it! How would you feel if it was happening to you? Liz stands in the kitchen and deliberately watches a saucepan boil dry and burn almost beyond redemption. I am gone. I do not know it is happening. I haven't been able to prevent it because I haven't known she was planning to let it happen! It can be very frightening.

New day, new paragraph. It is the 9th December 1996. Today I have decided that my psychiatrist is not normal. That is, if you define normality as

THE HUDDLE

conforming to the standards, attitudes, beliefs, hopes, behaviour etc. of the cultural majority in which you exist. You see, I have been conducting a quiet, discreet, undercover survey into what people *really* think about Christmas. I have watched and listened to Jan in work who has contact with many people, I have spoken to neighbours, I have eavesdropped at Tesco's and watched and listened on a recent shopping trip to Cardiff. The only adult I have heard confess they love Christmas is Dr. Kapp!! So that is not normal. She is not normal.

This discovery initially filled me with a flood of the most comforting smuggest relief! I was completely justified in my misery and dread of the coming Yuletide festivities because the rest of the adult population felt exactly the same way! Loads of us dreading it, looking upon it as a chore, reliving sad events and bereavements. Counting the cost and longing for the bloomin' so called jollifications to be over. So, silly psychiatrist for telling me to change the record, however difficult that might be, and enjoy Christmas for once! Why should I? It's more 'normal' not to!! It is now okay for me to be a miserable bloody pig and even own up to my state publicly and wallow in oodles of sympathy and swap stories with others about our seasonal gloom and depression. I am normal for once!!

But hang on…even I can see that there's something wrong about this. How sad an attitude! How terribly, horribly sad that so many people hate and dread Christmas. What has society done to Christmas that we are most of us in this state? Why should it be like this for so many? Why, God?

Janet Cooper

Why? Why is Christmas nothing but pain and sadness and cold and loneliness to so many? I mulled all this over, and Angel (Dr. Kapp?) spoke to me in the middle of my mind. "Dare to be different!" That's all she had needed to say to make me realise that with effort Christmas *could* be different for me this year and therefore so much more enjoyable for my family. I can't stop Christmas happening, but I can seek to change my attitude towards it! But how do I do that when my attitude towards it is as cold as ice?

"Dare to be different!" I could almost see Dr. Kapp smiling at me with question mark eyebrows which say, gently, "Well, what are you going to do about it then?" What indeed! I'll tell you what I'm going to do – I am going to turn into the category 'A' gold star patient that any psychiatrist would be proud to have. I am going to attempt, no, not attempt, I am *going* to do exactly what Dr. Kapp suggested during out last session together. That is, I am going to give some serious thought to all my bad feeling connected with Christmas. I shall have a jolly good cry over all the pain, the sadness, the loneliness, the memories and the hurts. Then I shall wrap them all up in brown paper, stow them or throw them away, and accept Dr. Kapp's permission to enjoy Christmas for once. I am going to give it a go, as there is nothing to lose and so much to gain.

If I can get through Christmas without wallowing in my own emotional muck, if I can be more unselfish and make it an enjoyable and exciting time for my family, if I can love more and have even

THE HUDDLE

a small inkling of the true spiritual significance of the birth of Jesus, then I shall be rich indeed!

WOW! Lord I believe. Help thou mine unbelief.

The Huddle, surprise surprise, already mock my intended efforts and whisper, whisper, whisper, reinforcing my suspicions that Dr. Kapp is tricking me by saying that she loves Christmas. They tell me that she doesn't really; she's only saying that she does because her training tells her to fill me with only that which is positive. Miserable voices! Miserable me! Dr. Kapp wouldn't lie to me! Would she? "Poor, trusting little cow…" Miserable, miserable, miserable Huddle! Please go! Please!!! In time for Christmas? Please? I am so very weary of them.

"Can me have a pressie?" Rachel has never had a Christmas present. My head too busy now. Stop typing then…

And yet how well I know this, because it has already started to happen. That if I decide to enjoy anything then The Huddle will get worse. The fight will intensify. It is more dangerous for me to be happy because they "hate me with a cruel hatred". They do not want my happiness, and so if I fight to enjoy Christmas I am either incredibly brave and courageous, or else I am a complete and utter fool to do something that will make me feel worse!!! The latter, I fear, must always be true. Does not scripture say that God has chosen the foolish things of this world to confound the wise? Are The Huddle wise? In a way, yes! They are wise to me. Wise to my every thought, word and action. Will I confound them by deliberately putting myself in their line of fire and claiming back a little of my potential to be a happy human being?

Hell and damnation to them!!! I HATE THEM!!!!!!!!!

Lord, silence please? If only for Christmas? I feel I would do *anything* just to have even *one* day without them.

Just one day? Please...

As I typed the last few paragraphs I was discussing The Huddle with Frank. "But I love Christmas, too!" He exclaimed. What? I was amazed! I have been married to him for over twenty years and never knew that he loved Christmas! How can that be? I thought he just got through it somehow, like I did. I can't remember any evidence that he actually enjoyed the festive season! How has he not been able to infect me with his love for this time of year? Is it because it was not obvious in any way? Is it because I would not let him? Is it because he's had to live with us? Me? Us?

Where was I? Oh yes. My psychiatrist. She also helps me to cope by allowing me to write to her, which I do quite frequently. This is incredibly therapeutic and cathartic, especially in the long, dark hours of a sleepless night. I believe I am able to better share the experience of being 'us' and having The Huddle if I do so in writing. I'm not a good talker, because when I talk I'm also hearing

THE HUDDLE

them, plus Rachel, but writing is different. It takes more concentration and I can see the words.

The letters to Dr. Kapp are usually long, maybe a dozen or more A4 pages, in which I tell her anything and everything. She so patiently reads every word, or so she tells me. Poor woman! It must be so boring! I write about The Huddle, going shopping, Rachel, housework, Jan, my cat, my kids, my past, Liz, Katy, Janny, what I'm wearing, what I ate for lunch, how I'm feeling and whether or not the cat has thrown up on the carpet etc.! Often I will begin by thanking her for our last session together and saying what I'd found relieving and helpful. Other times I will write to tell her off, get angry, imply that she's round the twist and wrong about certain things, and even accuse her of trying to send me round the twist! She accepts it all; accepting me exactly as I am at any one time. Like Jesus does.

I am immensely grateful for the way in which Dr. Kapp receives my numerous epistles and yet I will torment myself, probably unnecessarily, by imagining that my letters are nothing but an imposition, plopping through her letterbox and contaminating her territory. Hence I never like to post one that will arrive on a Saturday unless I am selfishly desperate to feel in touch. Saturday is the weekend and time off from people like us. Me.

I guess I could write a journal instead of sending all these over long letters, but it would not be the same as knowing somebody was reading what I'd written and would give me feedback at some time. Journals don't give feedback in the same way!

It has also been good for Rachel to be able to write to Dr. Kapp when she wants to, although I find it distressing to be 'absent' when a letter is written and posted. I don't know if any of the others have written letters. Maybe they have. I can't remember Rachel or Dr. Kapp mentioning any to me.

I have not always liked my psychiatrist. At the beginning of my psychotherapy she frequently pointed out that I would almost definitely go through a period of hating her. (Who? Me??) "But we'll work through it." She said. I thought the possibility of me hating her was nil! After all, she was there to help me and surely couldn't do that if I ended up hating her! Because then I wouldn't let her in my house for goodness sake! According to fundamentalist Christian doctrine submitted to me by Reverend H., I should not hate. It is sin. It is wrong. Not done. So I must not end up hating Dr. Kapp. Simple.

The Reverend's counselling had reduced me to floods of tears while I confessed aloud to God my hatred of certain people and begged His forgiveness for this most dreadful sin lest I not be saved from eternal damnation in the lake of fire where the worm never dies. (Poor s*dding worm!) Thus indoctrinated I was mega smug in my belief that hating my shrink would never happen. I was most certainly above that sort of sin, and temporarily oblivious to the concept of pride coming before a fall!

As my psychotherapy proceeded I felt that at times Dr. Kapp was deliberately provoking me to anger.

THE HUDDLE

"You're angry." She would say. Quietly. Infuriatingly quietly!

"No I'm not!" I would snarl back.

"Yes. You are." God, this woman spoke so quietly! I'll kill her….

"NO! I'M *NOT* BLOODY WELL *ANGRY!!!!!!!!!!!*"

To prevent myself admitting this very real anger, which came along with the feeling that I *could* end up hating Dr. Kapp, I would be screaming desperately inside my head for Rachel to 'come out' and rescue me from this unacceptable situation. I would push her forward so that I did not have to appear angry or hateful.

I got to feel that it was some crazy, textbook part of any psychotherapeutic relationship to go through a period of hating one's therapist, so that you could experience anger and hate in a safe environment where these often destructive emotions could be dealt with positively and safely. Transference and all that. I don't know! But whereas a psychiatrist might well be trained not to be hurt and damaged by being hated, a patient has no training to enable them to cope with the utterly confusing emotions of suddenly ending up (provoked into?) hating somebody you have struggled hard to trust. You feel so very vulnerable and unsafe when you hate somebody you need. Completely at their mercy. Very difficult. Very painful and confusing.

Anyway, it took quite a while for me to hate Dr. Kapp! It finally happened after fifteen months of weekly sessions and with me weighing six stone nothing. I absolutely hated her, I couldn't stand the sight of her, and I wanted to put my hands around her throat and twist her head back to front! How did this come about? Well, she arrived one day looking and acting decidedly ratty, and refused her usual cup of tea. She'd never refused a cup of tea before and so I was immediately on red alert. She sat down and proceeded to give me a right telling off about my weight.

"It's appalling! Whatever I do, whatever I say, you're not going to eat!" I sat there quietly, trying desperately not to cry. That day I had felt like the world's greatest success story because I hadn't *lost* any weight that week. But that wasn't going to be good enough. My weight was "Appalling! Appalling!"

Unfortunately, quirky anorexic that I was, I understood her to be saying that *I* was appalling, and so after that session I wrote her a note telling her that she wasn't doing me any good by speaking to me like that and I didn't want to see her ever again. We ended up having a break of exactly five weeks, which seemed forever after having had weekly sessions for over a year. I must have cried every one of those days, hating myself for what I'd done. Dr. Kapp had said at the beginning of my therapy "Whatever you do, even if you end up hating me, I will still come…." But she hadn't. And it was my fault, just as everything else bad that had happened to me was my fault. I had done something terrible.

However, I was also determined to show the silly old bag that I could manage without her. (I couldn't at that stage, but no way would she ever know that!) I still couldn't face much in the way of

THE HUDDLE

food, but miserably forced down cans of high calorie complete nutrition drinks. Yuk! They often made me sick. Then when I knew she was coming back (Frank had contacted her in an effort to negate my 'shove off' letter. I was too proud!) I was like a whirling dervish, making sure everywhere was neat and tidy, having a bath, doing my hair (what there was of it) and putting on clothes which I thought would make me look plump and healthy. On with a bit of make-up, practice a cheerful, nonchalant salutation, and bingo! All ready to resume my therapy where we had left off.

But it wasn't to be like that. She came. She went.

"I'll see you again in a month."

(A month? But I'd been seeing her every week!)

"Okay." I said. "That's fine. Thanks."

Conveniently forgetting I'd managed for five weeks without her, I went into panic mode. A MONTH?? Dr. Kapp wanted me to go on pretending to be okay for a whole, long, endless month? How? I could hardly see into next week! A month did not exist!

I felt this was my punishment. I was being punished for my anger, hate and nastiness and therefore I hated myself even more. I turned it all in upon myself and became very depressed, bricking Rachel up inside a bare cell and getting bogged down with The Huddle. I started cutting myself again but keeping it secret. Suicidal thoughts were real and constant.

So I did not cope with hating my therapist in any positive way. I see it as a destructive episode and look back on it as the most painful part of my psychotherapy.

Nevertheless, from Dr. Kapp's point of view, there was method in her madness and something good did eventually emerge from all this. I managed to get my weight up to seven stone (I'll show her!!) and only once since then has it dropped below this. Did Dr. Kapp mean for it to happen this way? Maybe, at the time, it seemed like the only way; upsetting me to save my life. I don't know. Was I really so very stubborn, awkward and unreachable? Was I really almost irreversibly on the road to starving myself to death? It would have been so easy to have done that. But I had hated somebody I had needed, liked and trusted. That was terrible and I still see it as very wrong. Feel so sad about it. Have to change the subject now.

Seeing as this is a chapter all about coping methods, do you want to know how I'm coping with The Huddle at this very minute? Even if you don't, I'm still going to tell you! They are in my desk lamp.
"F**king right we are, dull bloody bitch..."
They still do not want me to write this book and it has been getting harder and harder to sit at the typewriter and concentrate adequately for any length of time. So I have put on my earphones and I'm listening to music as I type. I listen to that and think about what I'm typing and that tunes me out of the voices, putting them into the background. It is also inclined to make my headache worse, but this is a small price to pay for being able to continue doing something *I* want to do! I am listening to a

THE HUDDLE

c.d. of Christmas songs which I bought along with a copy of J.S.Bach's St. John's Passion. Bloomin' brilliant stuff! At the moment I'm listening to Cliff Richard singing "Little Town". One line makes me cry,

"How silently, how silently the wondrous gift is given…"

It's the word 'silently'. Because I do not have silence. They are at me all day! Foul voices! But I am fine at the moment. Concentrating on these sentences, on hitting the right keys, on listening to the music, on staying tuned out of their miserable spoiling of my life.

"Me write my book, too, after?" Rachel. Well. Maybe. How? Can you type?

"Of course I can bloody well type!"

Slowing down now. Must rest before next paragraph…

Later. After a bit of a rest and a think, probably the best way to explain how I employ coping methods on a day to day basis would be to work through an example of a fairly typical day. Maybe a week day when I'm alone at home, and a day when I haven't just finished a ten hour night shift. So let's get going then!

I wake up, "Bitch is awake!" and before I plunge to the bottom of a pit of self pity and despair at having The Huddle with me for another day, I will almost always immediately get up. It is nigh on impossible to ever have even a short lie in with The Huddle around. I've tried it and I cannot do it. I cannot be their captive audience this way.

Janet Cooper

There is then the hustle and bustle busyness of getting breakfast and seeing Frank off to work and the kids off to school. This keeps my mind busy, but,

"We'll f**king get you girlie ... we can wait ... she gonna be all on her little wittle tod ... get you soon girl ..."

And so when everyone has left home, usually by 8.30am, I race up the stairs, two at a time, and quickly change into a pair of leggings and a t-shirt. I hustle back downstairs as if there isn't a moment to spare, The Huddle following furiously in the space around my head, and I work out energetically to a video tape. The Huddle will then settle into the butterfly I told you about previously. They will settle thus into an object when they know I'll be staying in one area for any length of time. This leaping aerobically around my room like a lunatic is extremely effective at getting The Huddle into the background at the beginning of the day when it is important not to let them immobilise and depress me. It is easy not to take notice of them when I am listening to energetic music, watching equally energetic fellow lunatics leaping about on my television screen, concentrating on my moves and getting out of puff. Wonderful! Vigorous exercise also, even after a sleepless night, perks me up somewhat and makes me feel all smug and healthy. It puts me in the mood for fighting The Huddle! Makes me stronger against them both mentally and physically.

After this exercise routine I will have a shower, concentrating all the time on what I am doing. I will

THE HUDDLE

think about the smell and feel and colour of the soap.

"Rubbing herself with f**king sh*t!"

I listen to the sound of the water spraying out of the shower and running down the bath.

"Bleeding on her ... covered with blood ... she see the blood coming out ... washed with the blood of sweet f**king Christ!"

I try to enjoy a brisk rub down with a towel, thinking about its colour, getting dry, and how nice it is to feel clean, if only temporarily.

"Go touch yourself, fat frigging cow!"

As well as super concentrating on anything I am doing, I will also start up a sort of mantra to fill my head with. It can be something as simple as 'the soap smells good, the soap smells good, the soap smells good', or something spiritual like 'be still, hear God, be still, hear God, be still, hear God'. Or, very easily and simply, I repeat the name 'Jesus'.

Rachel very often employs a sort of prayer mantra. She started doing this after Dr. Kapp wrote down a 'Jesus prayer' for us. Rachel repeats, sometimes for hours at a time, 'Lord Jesus Christ, have mercy on me a sinner'. Does this sound a bit gloomy and over serious for a seventeen year old? No. I don't think so. Why should it be? It calms her down. I can hear her when she does it and far from bothering me in a negative fashion, I find it very moving.

Some afternoons I give over to Rachel and find her sitting cross legged on the floor repeating this little prayer whilst fondling the beads of a rosary Dr. Kapp passed on to me. Jealous that I'd had a gift and she hadn't, Rachel pinched it from me and hid it away. It was only a few months ago, when we were beginning to be friendlier towards each other, that she gave it back to me and we arranged that we would share it. Rachel likes to cuddle its depiction of Jesus so that He is no longer a piece of metal hanging on the end of a string of beads, He is prayerfully real. She is cuddling and kissing the real Jesus.

Owing to my exorcism, occult interests and narrow minded evangelical indoctrination, Rachel's activities would once have horrified and sickened me, but not now, because God knows. He understands what's in our hearts and if Rachel comes to Jesus via a prayer mantra and a crucifix, then that's okay by Him. It would not have been okay with Rev.H, but he wasn't and isn't God, and doesn't know God as Rachel and I know Him. Dr. Kapp, being a Christian, has been able to teach us so much and we're so grateful to her. She has been a most wonderful 'spiritual director'.

After my shower I go into my bedroom to get dressed and this can be awkward. Rachel and I try to decide together on what will be worn that day while The Huddle remind us of what we are and are not allowed to wear. They don't like us, me, wearing anything white or pretty, preferring dark, drab colours. White underwear is allowed only because it will be covered up hopefully by something dark. I've recently started deliberately defying them be wearing bright, pretty colours, but they don't like it one bit. I have also perfected the art of dressing at top speed in order to better ignore their stupid commands and comments. Whilst I am dressing I will have the radio on in the bedroom in

THE HUDDLE

order to give myself something else to listen to other than The Huddle.

Radio still going, I'll then make the beds, or often Rachel will do this, me being absent and not knowing it's being done until I 'come back' and find out that it's done! "Me did that!" She will announce proudly. We used to argue a lot about this because she makes the beds in a different way to me and I wanted them made the way I like them made, with the pillows on top of the bedspread and not underneath. Now I realise that this sort of thing really does not matter and wasn't worth the aggro of getting mad about.

My morning will be spent doing the housework, which I enjoy, even though I believe my house shows little evidence of the effort spent on it! There are plenty of dusty corners, I've very conveniently forgotten how to hoover under beds and behind chairs, and if you open any cupboard then the contents will spill out to greet you.

My mother is somewhat house-proud, my sister is somewhat messy, and I am somewhere in between! I don't mind the kids rooms being untidy – these things are not important in the great scheme of things. The Huddle think differently and call me a lazy slovenly housewife. They say I am dirty and untidy. Even if that were true, so what? It is the untidiness of my mind that bothers me the most. It's too cluttered and too busy.

So. A morning of washing, ironing, cooking, cleaning and tidying around. All done to music and to the added accompaniment of an internal mantra. All watched and commented upon by The Huddle.

Janet Cooper

One thing I can get in a real tizzy about is wiping dishes. Firstly because I don't like handling knives, and secondly because I *have* to wipe up in groups of seven. That is, wipe seven items, put seven items away, wipe another seven items, put seven away etc. If I come to the end of the wiping up and there are exactly seven items left, then I am filled with the most ridiculous sense of joy, pride and relief. Success! I smile to myself and positively shudder with the sheer pleasure of having 'won'. If there are less than seven items left then it is not such an outright victory because I will have to find a few items in the kitchen to move or put away in order to make the number up to seven. I *know* this is daft, but it doesn't *feel* daft. I've tried to stop doing it but I'm well and truly hooked. Besides which, it's harmless!! It is not difficult to live with. Is it a compulsion or an obsession I wonder? I think I am stupid and of low intelligence.

When I am home alone (Alone? Ha ha, very funny!) I am allowed to sit down at exactly 11a.m. and have a cup of tea or coffee. Who allows me? I do! My drink will have to be stirred twenty one times in a clockwise direction, in three groups of seven. Seven because it's God's number and three because the Holy Trinity is three. Then it is safe to drink and the devil cannot turn it into blood, so no matter what The Huddle say, I will know that I'm not drinking blood. Again, I *know* this is daft, but it's the way I am, it's harmless, and it's unnoticeable to others. I have noticed that Jan in work will do the same – stir every drink with twenty one stirs and wipe up in sevens. Nobody takes the slightest bit of notice and it *doesn't* matter!!

THE HUDDLE

Well, yes, it *does* matter at times! It darn well annoys me and I wish I didn't *have* to do it. I become very frustrated with myself, failing to understand my stupidity, whilst also understanding that even these silly little compulsions are yet more ways of coping with The Huddle.

I am allowed to sit down for exactly twenty minutes and have my drink. It would be so wonderful to be able to sit quietly and gaze out of the window and think my own thoughts. Uninterrupted. Unsabotaged. But I cannot. If I did, The Huddle would grasp the opportunity to hurl themselves at me whilst my mind was not busy with anything specific. So while I have my drink I still need to keep my brain busy. I will read, write, or listen to music. What do I write? Maybe a letter to Dr. Kapp. A shopping list. This book.

I would say that music is my most effective method of tuning out of The Huddle. More so if I am listening via headphones which sort of symbolically exclude The Huddle from my ears all the while the music is filling my mind. Wonderful, wonderful music! If it's a bad Huddle day then I will sit, pressing the headphones hard to the side of our head, and rock myself backwards and forwards while I concentrate hard on the music. Often the tears will stream down my face, because the voices are vile and hateful, but the music, usually Bach, Mozart or Vivaldi, is so beautiful and profoundly moving.

Very occasionally during any day when The Huddle are really getting me down, I will sit and consciously tune *into* them, listening hard to everything they are saying. Sound crazy? Frank thought so when I first told him that I did this. He was horrified and feared for my sanity! But it can work, by me saying to them,

"Okay! You've got my undivided attention for the next fifteen minutes, I'm all yours, say what the hell you like, I'm listening! THEN!!! You jolly well leave me ALONE for a while!!!!"

This can get me tuned out of them for a number of hours but I need to be feeling brave to do this because it's not pleasant! The odd times when it *hasn't* proved effective, I've had great difficulty 'coming out of' the voices and have had to revert to my headphones double quick and double loud.

To understand how this 'tuning in' can work, I think of therapists who put arachnophobics in a room with spiders! They come face to face with what scares the life out of them in the hope of overcoming their fear and being able to cope with something that usually drives them batty! This *can* work! Am I explaining myself clearly and logically? Don't know. Don't care. Doesn't matter.

After the eleven o'clock cuppa there will be more pottering around the house until it is lunch time, when I will eat two slices of toast. On one slice I will have one low fat cheese triangle. This piece of toast then has to be cut into two triangles. The other slice is spread with either jam or honey and will be cut into two oblongs. I have to eat the oblongs first. Always when I am eating I have to do something else at the same time so as not to be sickened by what The Huddle say about food. They are very capable at stopping me from eating and my anorexic tendencies would make it so easy for me to go along with them. This 'something else' will

THE HUDDLE

either be reading, listening to music, writing, watching television, or, best of all, if the kids are home, sitting at the table and chatting. It is impossible to simply sit, eat and enjoy; food, therefore, has become very boring to me. Food is fuel and I eat because I've agreed to stay alive. And I feel bloomin' awful if I don't eat!

I once went out for lunch with my psychiatrist. I was feeling rather excited and special about this until I realised that there was no music, it would be extremely rude to read a book, toast was not featured on the menu and I couldn't think of anything to talk about! Rachel didn't care! She wanted a tuna and mayonnaise roll which duly arrived along with a beautiful salad and I let the willing and eager Rachel come forward and enjoy her feast. She ate our lunch for me – a little of it anyway! I don't remember eating it and I'm not sure if Dr. Kapp realised what was happening as she was busy herself enjoying a delicious looking meal of which I felt quite jealous. I would not have been able to eat the same and had chosen the safest, most allowed item from the menu. Rachel told me the roll, what she ate of it, was yummy, but she was too full to eat a much wanted ice-cream! As you can see yet again, my other personalities are also coping and defence mechanisms in situations like this.

Rachel is extremely angry at me now over that last paragraph. She always is when I refer to her as a coping mechanism!

"I'm not a bloody coping mechanism! I'm *me*! ***MYSELF! I AM ME!!!!!!!!!!!!!!!!***"

Janet Cooper

Okay, okay! I hear you! I take your point! I'm sorry, okay?

Thinking about food now, the thought of eating with a knife in one hand and a fork in the other is anathema to me. I do not like handling knives. I've already told you why this is, plus the mental pictures of slashes all over my body. I could not bear to hold a knife for the duration of a meal. But this in itself shouldn't stop me from eating a 'normal' meal! It's perfectly possible to eat with only a fork, but I still couldn't eat a 'normal' meal, as so many foods are not allowed and safe for me. Maybe the combination of The Huddle and having been anorexic have worked together in my mind to make food such a difficult issue for me, and although my diet is very restricted, I do eat enough of what I'm allowed. My weight is now stable and reasonable for my height (according to me!) and I am even able to admit to getting hungry now, which I wouldn't have done at one time. It's as if it's wrong for me to want to eat because it keeps me alive and therefore also feeds The Huddle. Also because they constantly tell me I am fat and gross and a glutton. Also because they turn my food into bones (toast), semen (yogurt), penises, testicles, foetuses, s**t (fruit), and stewed maggots (porridge). Porridge is a more recent addition to my diet. Have I already told you that? Doesn't matter.

Worms again.

Later. There were worms so I stopped typing.

THE HUDDLE

Then my beautiful children arrived home from school, my son so very proud, and rightly so, as he tells me of his 94% result for a maths test. My daughter so fizzy and excited because a friend has come to stay for the weekend. The two girls are now out carol singing, Frank has gone to visit a disabled friend and my son is playing on his Sega Megadrive. At least I think that's what it's called! So I can carry on typing. Clack, clack. A coping mechanism. Clack, clack. I can say what I like. Or can I??????

The cat is curled up asleep on a chair and I have my headphones on listening to Christmas music – to get me in the mood because Christmas will be different for me this year. The Huddle are in the desk lamp.

DAMN THEM!!!!!!!!!!

Okay then, worms gone and family fed and happily entertained – so on with the telling of a typical day!

With my little lunch out of the way I have a few more hours to get through before my children arrive home from school at about 3.30p.m. Sometimes I will go into town for library books. If I was not desperate to always have a book on the go then I would prefer not to make this journey as I hate the library. There are people there, shuffling quietly from aisle to aisle, from shelf to shelf, there are whispery voices and The Huddle whispering around my head. There are hands reaching out for books (or reaching out to grab ME???)

I will always be in a hurry to choose my books so that I can make my usual dash to the toilet which is two floors up from the library. Newport library is more effective than a dose of Senokot and always gives me the runs, I guess because of my anxiety and nervousness. Going into town is enough of an ordeal, but throw in a library visit and the torment is compounded.

Or rarely, instead of going to the library, I will go for a walk through the 'Squirrel Wood'. It's a delightful area near where I live and we've named it 'Squirrel Wood' because, yes, you've guessed (wasn't hard for goodness sake!), it's full of squirrels. It's such a pretty walk but lately I've been too depressed to enjoy it and take pleasure in the trees, flowers and little animals. That's a pity as it used to be so lovely for me. The Huddle have a lot to answer for!

Most often, after lunch, I will stay at home and these few hours before the kids arrive usually end up as time for my others. I do not willingly become absent and 'give over' to one of them. It just happens. Is there a part of me somewhere that allows it to happen? I must know, deep down, that I need to give them all some time, and besides which, it's a bit of a rest, me not being there. Or it can be. Mental anaesthesia. Yet 'me' cannot be completely out of control because I will always be 'me' again in time to prepare tea for the kid's arriving home. Rachel, I know, is aware that I have to see to the 'kiddiewinkies' and will always be gone back in time for me to do that. But the others? Janny is only three. I can return to find 'myself' playing with a bunch of cuddly toys which live in my

THE HUDDLE

living-room. It will never be later than three 0'clock! Or I can find myself standing, staring at another burned saucepan. It will never be later than three o'clock. Or I can find myself curled up on the floor or in a chair, hugging myself and either crying or close to tears. I can experience incredible pain and distress   until I realise what has happened and – Oh! – it's me again! Quick glance at the clock. It will never be later than three o'clock.

How on earth do the younger ones know how to time themselves? I don't remember these absences and as far as I am aware I do not consciously plan for them to happen – I don't like them as they make me very uneasy. Is it a case of me wanting so strongly to forget them, that I do? Am I really, totally absent at these times? If so, how am I always back again by three o'clock? Janny would not be able to tell the time. Or, and I have often wondered this, am I not the dominant personality who has control over all of us? Is it Jan who is the major person? Does she know exactly what is going on at any one time and thus able to organise time for all of us? Is she present at times when me, Frank, or anyone else doesn't realise it's her? Why am I only aware of her in work? I don't know. So many questions and so few answers.

Most people do shorten my name to 'Jan' but I do realise that they mean me, Janet, and not the real Jan. Dr. Kapp only recently started to shorten my name to Jan and this did initially confuse me because I am used to her talking to the others and initiating this by calling them by name. Did she want to talk to Jan? My nasty, suspicious little mind has wondered if she called me this to see if Jan would speak to her. Maybe Jan did speak to her. I don't know. Now I've got used to Dr. Kapp calling me, Janet, Jan. Confused? It isn't confusing, really it isn't. It makes so much sense for me to be as we are.

So my kids come home. It is wonderful when they arrive back from school! They rush in like a breath of fresh air and I am immediately taken up with all their news about the day.

"Mad Mike was on the bus again Mum!"

"Guess what Mum, right, Jamie fancies me!"

I sit at the table with them and eat toast and chat while they enjoy an early dinner. They are always ravenous when they arrive home from school and I don't see the point of making them wait for a meal until later. After food, their friends will phone or call, there's homework to be done, schoolbags to sort out and cartoons on the television to sit and watch together, all cuddled up on the settee. Their wonderful, precious company helps me to cope with The Huddle but I will never ever refer to my children as a coping mechanism. They are so very much more than that. Brilliant, lively, wonderful, unique, fascinating, and special people. I love them so much and detest the fact that my 'malady' causes them distress.

When the kids have been home for about an hour I will nearly always need to tune out of The Huddle again for a while. The voices get desperate for attention and almost jealous when I am with my kids.

DAMN THESE VOICES TO HELL!!!!!!!

THE HUDDLE

So either on with the headphones or out with a book! Sadly, my children are used to me becoming vague and unhearing before doing this. If I am not able to read, then I will pretend to read so that my children will know to leave me alone while I then 'tune out' by chanting a mantra or going through music inside my head. It must be so awful for my children when I act as if I'm not taking much notice of them. I will arrive at the point where I am finding it difficult to concentrate on what they are saying – it's like they are trying to speak to me in the middle of a noisy crowd. Both kids are used to Janny making her funny little noises, and Rachel sharing their playground humour by being silly and giggly. It's just Mum being a bit daft! But there *has* to be a controller among us (Jan? Angel?) because I have never noticed Janny squeaking like a constipated hamster when my kids have their friends around. These friends are also used to seeing me typing, writing, headphones on, engrossed in book – It's just how it is and children can be so much more accepting than adults!! Sometimes when my neighbour calls and I am busy like this, he will accuse me of not wanting to talk to him and being a 'miserable swine today'! But he knows about the voices, and this is his way of coping with a vague, silent and seemingly ignorant me. It's more acceptable to call me a miserable swine than acknowledge that my voices are bad!

My children know about The Huddle but they know very little about the others, only that I feel as if I have little girls inside me who cry a lot and are very sad. My kids know as much about my condition as I feel they are able to understand and accept, and I answer their questions as honestly as I can, taking into account their ages. They know that Dr. Kapp is a psychiatrist and that psychiatrists treat people with mental illnesses, but they find this a bit puzzling! They don't see me as 'mental'. Neither do I!! I am their mother, they don't know what other mothers are like, and they accept me and love me as I am. Obviously they get upset at times when I am depressed and silent, it isn't easy for them, but every day, without fail, I will tell each of them that I love them. "I love you so much". Even when I was severely depressed and didn't speak for months I still managed to mouth those words to them, and if I couldn't even manage this, I would write them on pieces of paper to give to them. At a time when I believed and felt that I was incapable of loving, this was an enormous effort, but one which I am so glad and thankful I was able to make.

Evenings in our house are generally very busy. There might be the twice weekly visit to the supermarket, always the kids are in and out with their mates, expecting an endless supply of food and drink for growing bodies, and at intervals throughout the evening I'll need to dive into one of my coping mechanisms. I don't cope well with several human voices and/or the television for any length of time as it makes The Huddle more confusing. So I will play the piano, type, read, or back to the good old headphones. Often I will curl up in a chair and close my eyes. This means 'leave me alone for a while as I need to tune out of my voices'.

Frank tends to snap 'leave your mother alone!' if the kids disturb me like this, but thankfully I've

THE HUDDLE

managed to stop him doing this. It just makes it worse for me and the kids, and I am still capable of communicating to them in some way while I'm distant and vague. I feel so sorry for them having a mother like me! It must be horrible.

"What are the voices saying, Mam?"

"Oh, they're swearing at me as usual and telling me I'm stupid."

"Tell them to get lost!"

Oh! I have done!! So many times!!! Truly I have done…….

When the kids have gone to bed Frank and I might play Scrabble. He very rarely wins! I often accuse him of letting me win in order to make me feel better about myself, but he assures me, somewhat indignantly, that this is not the case! He wishes it was true, but it isn't!! It is very odd that if I am well tuned out of The Huddle I will still win at Scrabble, but only just. Yet if they are really getting me down and I'm totally fed up, frazzled and fuzzyheaded from headache tablets, then up zooms my score and Frank doesn't stand a chance! This could be because of the extra concentration needed to do anything when the voices are bad. Another explanation might be that at times I make greater efforts *because* I have The Huddle; that is, an enemy to fight against.

That leads me on to other questions. Like, would I be an even more pathetic excuse for a human being if I *didn't* have The Huddle to fight against on a daily basis? Would I collapse into a permanent rotting depression and cease making any effort to survive? This would imply that I need The Huddle in order to survive as a reasonably functioning organism and I simply don't hold with that! I need them like I need a hole in the head, and imagine myself as being so much better off if I did not have them. These are provoking trains of thought which I generally prefer not to give room to. Disabled people may well curse their disabilities and yet many lead amazingly useful and successful lives. Is this because they have a disability to fight against? Yet others collapse under the burden of it all. Life is very strange. I can make no sense of it.

The nights that Jan does not go into work are a misery for me. If I do manage to sleep then it will only be for a few hours. I've already written about my sleepless nights so I won't bore you further by repeating myself.

"Good! Thank God for that!" (That's Rachel)

Frank has recently acquired some different sleeping tablets for me to try but unfortunately these don't work either and simply leave me feeling groggy and unpleasant the next day, and with a foul taste in my mouth. Medication has never been a very useful coping mechanism for me and I have tried enough of it over the years.

I am actually producing these very words at 4a.m. in the morning. It is a bitterly cold night, and the fire flickers, causing the tinsel on the Christmas tree to shimmer and sparkle. It is pretty, and I can actually *see* that it is pretty! How wonderful! The cat keeps pestering me to give her a bit of a fuss, one of the hamsters is squeaking, my tea has gone cold and The Huddle are in the desk lamp. They are watching me, always watching me, typing away and they are absolutely furious that I am taking no

THE HUDDLE

notice of them yelling their foul, boring, pathetic obscenities at me. They keep telling me to rip this book to shreds. I am not going to do that.

I feel very, very tired and fed up. Do you know what I'd like to do right this very minute? Ring my G.P., get him up out of his warm, cosy bed, and shout at him,

"For God's sake give me something to make me sleep! I can't stick it! Why won't you give me something that will get rid of it all? Do you hate me as well? Help me......."

But I know that he can't give me anything that will get rid of The Huddle and the others. Because there isn't anything. I feel hopeless about it all. Here I am, chatting away to you, and I don't even know who you are!

Later on... In fact it is now evening and J.S.Bach's Christmas oratorio is coming gloriously through my headphones. Beautiful music to drown out The Huddle! They struggle to superimpose themselves over it.

GO AWAY! PLEASE!!!!!!!!!!!!

I did eventually go back to bed this morning and finally fell asleep, waking up at quarter to ten ('Bitch is awake!') in the middle of a peculiar dream. I'd been dreaming that Frank had thrown all our furniture out of the back window and into the garden. He was furiously hacking it to bits. I asked him why he was doing this and he told me that everything was a mess and he couldn't stand it. I replied that it was only the Christmas decorations that were making everything a bit untidy, but that it didn't matter. He had also ripped down all the curtains and put sheets and blankets up over the windows. Dr. Kapp arrived and I was trying to tell her what he was doing but she was acting as if she couldn't see anything wrong and I was making a fuss about nothing. The hamster and gerbils had been let out of their cages and a strange dog was in the kitchen eating the cat's food. The kitchen floor was absolutely filthy.

So I'd woken from this odd dream and, as usual, The Huddle were watching me from their place in the window. I got up immediately, came straight downstairs and had two pieces of toast. I cut one into triangles and…. Then Frank made tea.

"Did you stir it properly?"

"Yes love, I did. Twenty one times."

But did he? And had he done it in three groups of seven stirs? Was he just telling me he'd done it when really he hadn't? It was to be yet another day of it all! Another bloody day, excuse my language. But today I was clever and had scored an early victory by putting on my pretty white blouse!

"Don't you **DARE** wear that **THING!!**"

"Oh sod off and leave me ALONE!!!"

"Tut-tut! Language! Naughty, naughty!"

One coping method I've not yet discussed is yoga. This can be brilliant, but only when I'm already coping pretty well. My ability to do yoga is affected by whether or not I have taken any medication and what I have taken. When I was

THE HUDDLE

taking Largactil regularly my balance and concentration was not good and unfortunately rendered this gentle exercise almost impossible and therefore ineffective. Also, yoga is a very quiet and peaceful activity and The Huddle find it easy to infiltrate my attempts at stillness and tranquillity. But sometimes yoga *can* work and when it does I am left most wonderfully relaxed and refreshed.

Other methods I have tried include aromatherapy, writing music, drawing, deep meditation, prayer, saturating myself with scripture, going to church, various medications and the laying on of hands by a self professed healer. All had varying degrees of success and failure. One might work for one day, but not the next, but at least these were harmless and potentially enjoyable pursuits.

My most destructive 'coping mechanisms' have included anorexia, cutting all my hair off, self mutilation, exorcism, invocation of the spirit world, trying to turn my back on God, planning and attempting suicide, and the constant and always present temptation –'if you can't beat 'em, join 'em'! How? Well, If I went back to all the secrecy of the occult then I would be joining The Huddle, so they tell me, and they would love me to do that. They want it to happen and keep promising me peace if only I will do this one thing and again share a tyrant of a master with them.

Would I have peace? Maybe for a few weeks while The Huddle deluded me into thinking I'd made the right decision, but then they would flood back into my life and my last state would be worse than my first. Besides which, I know it would be wrong. Evil. A sin. Better the devil you know? Not for me, thankyou, I've tried him and he did me no good. Look at the mess I am in! I shall instead continue my fight to know Jesus because somehow I just *know* that He must be worth it. He is gentle, lovely and kind. The Huddle are not.

This temptation to join The Huddle instead of fighting against them is very real and very distressing to me because it *is* so tempting! Peace for even one day can seem worth anything at all. In fact, peace for an hour would make me think I'd landed in paradise! 'Don't do it! Please don't go back!' Says Angel (Dr. Kapp?), and I know that I mustn't.

"Neither give place to the devil. Let him that stole steal no more. (Ephesians 4:27, 28) "And have no fellowship with the unfruitful works of darkness, but rather reprove them." (Ephesians 5:11)

But...

My psychiatrist is aware of this struggle and plans to help me deal with it. Not sure how. Maybe I could prayerfully turn these awful temptations and thoughts into a 'thing', like a spirit of witchcraft that clings to me and tries to drag me backwards all the time. Then I could prayerfully 'dump' this thing as I did my evil comforter. It could work. It will work. It *has* to work! Then maybe when I have done that The Huddle will go??????????

I've just had a thought! Would it be correct to describe my periods of depression as a coping

THE HUDDLE

mechanism, albeit a profoundly tormenting one? When I am really bogged down by The Huddle and life becomes too frantic to live from one coping method to another, do I retreat and escape from the struggle by becoming depressed? Just giving in and rotting. Not having to cope. Not having to speak or do anything. Not having to care about how much they are tormenting me. Not having to care what the bloody hell happens to me. Not having to feel, or love, or smile or pretend. Just crash down and out for a while. Be dead and rot. Let the damn things have me, what the hell do I care? I've nothing to live for anyway. Just be dead and not care…

I cannot say that my mustard seed faith is a coping method although I wish with all my heart that I could. The Huddle are at their most vicious in their fight against Jesus and anything to do with Him. I have been able to soar to splendid heights when reading hymns and scripture, feeling and knowing a wonderful connection to Jesus, but these flights are so very rare! Therefore all the more precious because of their infrequency. The most usual scenario is that The Huddle make it such a misery to follow my chosen Christian faith that I consider myself prayer-less and oft times without the courage to enter the battle that is necessary if I am to read and inwardly digest the scriptural words and verses I have come to love so much. Why does God not make it easier for me? Why is it so hard for me to follow Jesus? Why don't I just give up, become a Buddhist, or a Mormon, or a bloomin' pagan and save myself an awful lot of trouble and misery? The thing is, you don't give up someone you love who is good for you! I've tried often and hard to give Jesus up, but I can't. Being so opposite to Satan and to The Huddle is what makes Jesus so irresistible and everything I want. Yes, I am often tempted to hurtle off in the opposite direction, but then so was Jesus Himself! It is not a sin to be tempted!

I want to see Jesus and I want to see heaven. "There shall be no night there; and they shall need no candle, neither light of the sun; for the Lord God giveth them light." (Revelation 22:5) "And God shall wipe away all tears from their eyes, and there shall be no more death, neither sorrow nor crying, neither shall there be any more pain, for the former things are passed away." ((Revelation 21:4)

I have been cruelly indoctrinated with belief in a literal hell.

"Unless you are delivered, Janet, then we fear you will go to hell." Said Reverend H and his wife. By 'delivered' they meant not hearing voices. Reverend H spoke to my other personalities and told them to go to hell.

"Out! In the name of Jesus, and go to the pit where you belong! We hate you, God hates you, the whole of heaven hates you! GO! OUT!!!"

You can imagine the state we were all in after two years of this! We were all terrified. Some of us still are! We are not recovered from this albeit well meant abuse. Scripture was used against us, hymns were sung to torment us, hell was always before us, and the devil was laughing his bloody head off!! Reverend H showed me Jesus in all His glory, then snatched Him away from me, substituting a severe and punishing God who would not tolerate my undelivered state for ever. The Reverend might have meant well, but he was severe, ignorant about abnormal psychology and unwise to treat me without medical cover. He was also a very proud man. I wish with all my heart that I had never met him. So does Rachel. Katy and little Janny are still terrified of him. Any way, I digress…

I was on about hell. The Huddle are hell! I already exist on the fringes of a literal hell; I hear it every day! Hell is voices and darkness and rotting and misery. Jesus is not hell. He is calmness and light and health and joy – and I want Him! "Let me never be put to confusion, deliver me in thy righteousness and cause me to escape: incline thine ear unto me and save me." (Psalm 71:1,2)

I suppose I could go on and on explaining why I cling to the Christian faith, presenting countless arguments and quoting scripture. Maybe that would fill another book?

"NO!! You said I could do *my* book next!" (That's Rachel again. She's watching me type.)

But really, I can sum up my reasons in four words. <u>BECAUSE I LOVE JESUS!!!!</u> I have typed that in capital letters and underlined it in order to torment The Huddle.

"READ IT, DAMN YOU, READ IT!!!!!!"

I will continue with the coping mechanisms and I will continue with the fight. It's easy to say that when I'm not depressed! Fight! Fight! Because I have no choice. I hate it and I blame God for it. I get so angry with Him. I feel I am weak and ill equipped. But I cannot stop loving Jesus.

"For we wrestle not against flesh and blood, but against principalities, against powers, against the rulers of the darkness of this world, against spiritual wickedness in high places. Wherefore take unto you the whole armour of God, that ye may be able to withstand in the evil day, and having done all, to stand." (Ephesians 6:12) Go read it and read on, imaginary reader! It's brilliant stuff!

A sort of prayer – 'Lord, I *am* trying to cope. Please – You cope for me? Just for a day so that I may have silence. Put Your armour upon me and polish it shiny bright with the light of Christ that will repel them. Lord, please, please, please take The Huddle away from me. Please? If only for a day! "For a day in thy courts is better than a thousand. I had rather be a doorkeeper in the house of my God, than to dwell in the tents of wickedness." (Psalm 84:10)

"My soul longeth, yea, even fainteth for the courts of the Lord. My heart and my flesh crieth out for the Living God." (Psalm 84:2)

I shall not be dismayed.
I SHALL FIND GOD!

THE HUDDLE

CHAPTER EIGHT   DRUGS

"…in vain shalt thou use many medications; for thou shalt not be cured." (Jeremiah 46:11)

This line conjures up memories of Reverend H when he used to insist that drugs and psychiatry could not help me.

"*I can help you, Janet!*" How arrogant! Whenever I was in the grip of one of my awful depressions, rather than suggest I should go to my doctor, Mrs. H would often quote to me, "The dog returneth to his vomit." (Proverbs 26:11) and the two of them would then attempt to exorcise my psychiatric demons. For example, the evil spirits of depression, psychosis, mania, schizophrenia, hysteria, madness, lunacy, confusion, anxiety, dementia etc. etc. The idea being, if I was delivered of these awful demons then I would be 'better' and not in need of any drug therapy or psychiatric help. I was to rely on God (via the Reverend) and nothing else. (Amazing to be full of so many terrible demons and still work and care for my family!!)

However, exorcism did not un-rape me, heal any of my emotional wounds or cure any depression. In fact it made everything a great deal worse, significantly adding trauma to trauma. I would say with confidence now that a lot of my symptoms during this period of exorcism were iatrogenic, that is, caused by my 'therapist', the Reverend. Little wonder that I ended up slightly round the twist and in St. Cadoc's.

Janet Cooper

There was, however, some truth in what Reverend H said about drugs not being able to help me, even though they have only ever been prescribed in the hope of alleviating my distressing symptoms. I wish there was something I *could* take that would help me cure my depressions and get rid of The Huddle. I no longer know if I *want* to get rid of the others as we are so used to being this way and all my attempts to rid my life of them have failed. Maybe we are meant to be as we are and the best thing to do is to get used to it again, and get on with each other like we did before the Reverend H arrived on the scene. What the hell else can we do anyway?

At the very moment a prescription for Stelazine languishes in the local pharmacy awaiting my collection. I had read in the Reader's Digest about somebody who took this to get rid of their voices and it had worked. 'This is it! Why hasn't anybody told me about this drug that will get rid of The Huddle? Quick! Give me some! Give me lots of it!!' My G.P. sounded quite enthusiastic when Frank rang him about my miracle cure and thought it was at least worth a try. My psychiatrist was *not* so enthusiastic and thought that maybe it wasn't worth a try as it is a drug so similar to Largactil, which I've already been taking, that I would probably suffer the same unpleasant side effects that led me to come off Largactil a few weeks ago. Besides which, Dr. Kapp and I discussed that because of the way I'm feeling at the moment (totally piddled off and desperate), if I was to pin any hopes on this drug shutting The Huddle up, and it didn't, then the disappointment and let down would be devastating.

THE HUDDLE

My present mental state will not allow me the risk of this sort of disappointment; therefore I won't be collecting the prescription. Deep down I can't see, anyway, how medicating *me* will get rid of The Huddle. They are external to me, of that I am convinced. I have to be!

Yes, I suppose I'll always hang on to a feeling of 'I'll try anything', but only to a point. I've tried several drugs and none of them have been particularly helpful. All they've done is build up false hopes, only to have them tormentingly dashed after days, weeks and months of religiously swallowing the prescribed medication.

Drugs I can remember having taken at some time include Largactil (Chlorpromazine), Valium, Seroxat, Melleril, Molipaxin, Lofepramine, Loprazolam and Zimovane. The last two are sleeping tablets. The only two I have taken for any length of time are Lofepramine, an antidepressant, and Largactil, which is an anti psychotic tranquilliser. The only one that has been of any significant help at all is the Largactil, and yet surely it is The Huddle, and not me, that needs the anti psychotic, tranquillising effects!!

On the 22nd September 1995 I wrote this.
Rachel is in brackets.
The Huddle are in speech marks.
The music I was trying to concentrate on is in block capitals.
My writing and thoughts are in italics.
(Yeh! Complicated eh? Go on! Have a go at it......)

By the way, Rachel's language has improved dramatically since this was written.

A PRELUDE TO LITTLE WHITE PILLS

So Jan arrived home from work and I kissed my babies off to school and Frank off to work, snuggling into bed at 8.30a.m. I got up at 11.20a.m had toast, coffee, a little white pill and walked to town where I had a haircut.
Walked home. Showered to get the itchy bits off. Put on clean clothes. Made more toast and coffee and sat in my chair to read my library book. I couldn't. Concentration bad. Just can't do it. Tired. Headache. Feel a bit shaky. We still don't feel well.

(Your hair's too short, fat face!)

Get lost! Brick her up in her cell, block her out, brick her up, brick, brick, brick, brick…….
Silent screams.

(NO! Don't you DARE do that to me! You can't! Won't! Don't! I'm warning you! I'll cut you to f**king pieces you cruel bloody bitch! Don't you…)

I start to think I am going mad again.
Just get out of MY head, will you? OUT!!!!!

(P*ss off! I hate you, I hate you, I hate you, I hate you, I hate……)

Screams.

THE HUDDLE

"S**t! The cut slut had hair cut – Katy did, Katy did, Katy did – They're p*ssing well arguing again see gorgeous fat c**t she's looking – Katy did, Katy did, Katy did…"

I look at the butterfly where The Huddle are now coming from and I almost begin to cry.

"Knows we're talking about her, all times s**t rhymes – Katy did – fat cow can't read s**t book now, brown cow…"

(Well don't bloody well listen to them then! Mine are worse than yours anyway! I know more…)

Brick, brick, brick, brick, brick, brick, brick…

(Don't you bloody f**king DARE! You fat, cruel, s*dding bitch!!)

DOMINE FILI UNi…   (Vivaldi's 'Gloria')

"She can't read now! Put that book down NOW!!!!!!! Look, put book down, fat f**king cow and suck cock – Katy did, Katy did – can't read, on speed, Katy did…"

…GENITE JESU…

(I hate you, I hate you, I hate you, I hate you…)

"Katy did – she'll smash her face against the ba*tard wall and Aunty washes, dresses and gets out messes, mud on crud to p*ss on mud floor and cock sprays gorgeous little fat …"

…CHRISTE. DOMINE…

(I hate you! Cruel bitch, cruel bitch, cruel bitch, cruel bitch…)

"She eaty beaty hell toast and most hell roast she see Satan suck sweet Jesus, f**k the Jesus, sit on Christ to wank Him off and p*ss some more on floor and eat all blood and – Katy did, Katy did, Katy did – we know, we know, fat c**t slut cut hair more sore a*se…"

I think. Hard. Try to. Help me. Yoga? Play piano? Get busy? Scream? Kill myself?

(P*ss off! I'm not doing anything! I'm not well, don't feel well, won't do anything. Won't! Won't!!!)

"She won't. They don't. We won't. <u>KILL YOU'RE F**KING SELF AND PUT US ALL OUT OF THIS MISERY WHY DON'T YOU?</u> She kill her too but Rachel scared cow. She'll kill her and cut slut. They fight, no sight for Katy did, Katy did, Katy did – and out, out, out, in and out, in and out, in and out…"

Today I am not brave. I am tired. Today I want a rest. Today I do not want to have to cope. Cry? I'd rather die! It does not matter.
Be dead, be dead,
Escape this head,
And out and out she shouts, they shout,

THE HUDDLE

And I am her at whom they leer
And talk about and snigger,
Pull the trigger
On my life
Please!

All you that <u>really</u> love me
LET ME GO!!!!!

Actually I think that I may already be dead. Jan in work last night was exhausting. Feel very bitty and split off. We are not happy in my head today. You lot, please, please go away! I'm dead. Just a mass of cut off bits that scream and squirm. I want a rest. All I want to do is have a rest.
So I give in and give up.
Go take the little pills instead.
Two of them.
Chemical relief for poorly head.
And very soon I'm sluggish and I snooze.
Quieter now.
Till when?
And then?...

Later on now. The kids are home from school and my body is smiling and functioning. Me? Who the hell is 'me' anyway? Where am I?

Sarah, a friend from down the road, calls and tells me I don't look very well. I tell her I'm fine. Just tired. I work nights. Makes you a bit tired. That's all.

Frank arrives home from work.

"Had a good day, love?"

Janet Cooper

"Yes! Fine! Normal!"
Perfectly normal………………………..

I think this excerpt from my journal give a good example of the circumstances under which I will take Largactil, other than or additional to a regular daily intake. I take it when I am severely bothered and unable, or too tired, or too fed up to cope in other ways. Or maybe I have tried several other ways of coping but have failed.

Largactil will work by nearly knocking me out! Amongst other side effects, they make me feel heavy, slow, sluggish, lethargic, sleepy and indifferent. This means that my reception of The Huddle is blurred, their volume lowered, and I haven't the energy to take much notice of them. The trouble is, I haven't the energy to do much else either! The lethargy and sluggishness that these tablets produce is unpleasant and has to be experienced to be understood. But, and especially at night, it can be better than feeling that The Huddle will drive me mad. Largactil gives me a bit of a rest, albeit at a price, but the price is often worth it. A change can be as good as a rest, so I change one set of unpleasant stuff for another!

After taking Largactil, the time I would otherwise have spent coping with The Huddle will then become time spent dozing restlessly or curled up on the settee feeling too sluggish, lazy and indifferent to bother or want to do anything else. Therefore, from the point of view that the Huddle are a waste of time, I'm really no better off. I'm

THE HUDDLE

either forced to live frantically, from one method of coping to another, or else I'm drugged up. Either way I'm unable to do what *I* want to do when *I* want to do it!! Some choice! Do I feel a pity party coming on? Hope not…

For example, much as I love to sit and type, at the moment I'm suffering from a nasty cold and would like nothing better than to be able to sit in a chair, feet up, eyes closed, relax, be quiet and think about nothing in particular. But I can't! If I do not keep my mind constantly busy then The Huddle will torment me, so here I am furiously typing away and wondering if anybody on this crazy planet will ever read this crazy book about crazy me!!

Why not take some extra Largactil now? Because they make me feel so bloody awful, that's why! Upping the daily dose is for desperation points only or when time and circumstances permit. I can't indulge today because I have more Christmas shopping to do and my daughter has a friend staying with us, so I don't want to embarrass her by lurching around giddily under the influence of little white pills!

The thing is, I haven't got time to be coping with The huddle, and yet I damn well have to! Damn and blast them to hell!!

I DO NOT WANT THEM!!!!!!!!!!!!!!!!

Apart from dulling my reception of them and my reactions to them – which is certainly of use at times – Largactil does not actually affect The Huddle in any way. Well it wouldn't, would it? They are external to us. Me. It does not make them any less obscene, blasphemous or offensive. Neither does it slow down or slur their speech. It does not shut them up or make them go away. It makes them sound muffled, or as if they are a way off, in the distance, although I sense that they still occupy their usual spaces and follow me around. Pity The Huddle can't swallow the damn tablets instead of me! Now that would make far more sense!

Other side effects I experienced on a regular, four times a day dose were – dizziness, loss of concentration, increase in bad dreams, stuffy nose, feeling cold all the time, breast pain and discharge from the nipples, pains in my legs, sensitivity to light and the occasional fluttery heartbeat. At least, I've attributed these symptoms to Largactil. Gruesome list, eh? Thankfully most of these symptoms have cleared up now that I'm only taking the stuff as required – that is, when I'm desperate. Not taking them regularly throughout the day has meant that the voices, The Huddle, have seemed worse, or rather my reception of them has been unblurred, heightened and more acute. The pay-off is everyone telling me I appear brighter, more alert and with-it, and busier. I'm certainly busier! It's a case of having to be, but that's not necessarily a bad thing. It's meant, for a start, that I've begun writing this book which is proving incredibly therapeutic and cathartic, even though The Huddle will always try to make it seem otherwise.

There are times when I cannot take Largactil. I cannot take it within eight hours of working a night shift because Jan needs to be alert and energetic. I cannot take it when I need to go shopping or into town. I cannot take it if my kids have their friends

THE HUDDLE

round or during school holidays. (Although I have done – but prefer not to) It is not fair for my kids to have me dozing and slouching all over the place. It's far better for them to see me plugged into some music or typing furiously. Neither can I read, do yoga, exercise, play the piano or keep busy whilst under the influence of this drug.

So you see, although Largactil is a crutch to fall back on, it is not the sort of help I would choose on a day to day basis. I just hate the way it makes me feel and believe that I am better off taking it only when desperation dictates that I need to be knocked out for a few hours. But then, the awful, terrible dreams..... I wonder if Largactil actually produces these foul nightmares. Or is it a case of me being so drug-dozy that I cannot escape my dreams by waking up? Do I simply remember my dreams more clearly when on Largactil?

Tell you what; I'm getting bored writing about Largactil. Are you bored reading about it? Tough. My book!

Dr. Kapp has never prescribed medication for me. As she points out, her field is child psychiatry and therefore she is not suitably updated on the latest drugs and dosages for adults, and so has not wanted to be involved in any prescribing on my behalf. Sounds fair enough, I suppose. But what a flaming nuisance! Here I am, seeing a consultant psychiatrist on a regular basis over a period of years who refuses to prescribe any medication for me! I either have to see another (adult) psychiatrist or else go to my G.P., which is usually what I've done. It has infuriated me at times.

That is, until very recently, when Dr. Kapp *did* suggest some medication for me to try. Frank chatted to my G.P. about it, who strongly advised me not to take it, and when I looked up the side effects I was horrified! So I then wrote Dr. Kapp a nasty letter accusing her of not caring a damn and trying to poison me! So really it's just as well, in view of the fact that pills have not been much help to me, that she is *not* involved in prescribing me these dashed hopes! I would be blaming her and hating her all over the place and two 'I hate you' periods (five weeks, and nearly five months) are quite enough, thank-you! More than quite enough!!

It was early this year, towards the end of the longer 'I hate Dr. Kapp' period that I saw one of these other psychiatrists. She was, in fact, the third of the 'other' psychiatrists that I had seen. I had been dead against seeing her at all and I'll refer to her as Dr. D. because her surname began with a 'D'. Clever, eh? Anyway, it was Dr. Sami, my G.P. who had persuaded me to see her as I was still adamantly refusing to see Dr. Kapp, or allow him to contact her on my behalf. It came about thus –

I had sat in Dr. Sami's surgery in tears while he and his nurse saw to some nasty gashes on my back which had been inflicted by a very frightened, tormented and confused Katy. I had been scared to go to Dr. Sami again for help, fearing that he would be fed up with the frequency of all this cutting and bundle me off to casualty. So I'd waited, blood-soaked, until Frank could escort me down to the surgery. And escort me he certainly did. Angrily, tearfully and desperately.

"When's all this going to end, love? Tell me!"

THE HUDDLE

"When I'm dead." Well, I was probably only being honest!!

"You'll have to go into hospital if you keep on like this!" He was forever threatening to have me committed!

Thankfully and amazingly, Dr. Sami turned out to be his usual self when confronted with us and our gashes. He was wonderfully patient and gentle, but also very insistent that I needed help, and urgently. He ordered Frank not to leave me alone, and all tablets were to be kept out of my reach. He tried talking to me.

"Janet. This can't go on."

"It won't. I'll be dead soon."

"Why do you say that?"

"Because it's true! I've had enough, nobody can help me, I've tried everything so I'm going to kill us, I've made my mind up and I'm not going to change it...."

"Janet? Listen to me. I will ask Dr. Kapp to see you."

"No! I don't want to see her. She hates me!" I really believed it too! Dr. Sami was not to be put off!

"I will arrange for somebody else to see you then."

"NO!" I snapped. "There's no point, I've made my mind up, the only way out is to kill me, I'm just not sure when…"

"Janet!" Dr.Sami again. "Listen! You must not do this! You are a wife and a mother! You cannot…"

"They'd be better off without me!"

"No, Janet! They…"

And so the argument went on, until I realized that I should have kept quiet, and in order to get Dr.

Sami off my back I agreed, reluctantly, to see this other psychiatrist. I planned to be dead before she arrived. Unfortunately, Frank arranged for special leave from work and never left me for a second, even coming with me to the loo. Dr. Sami had pleaded with me not to do anything stupid. I never got the chance!

About two days later this Dr. D arrived. I had already decided that she wouldn't be able to help me because I didn't want to be helped. She was also younger than me which didn't help. I don't like people younger than me trying to be wiser than me *about* me! But I did manage to behave ourselves! I was very good, sat still, and talked to her. I told her that I planned to kill myself; my mind had been made up for some time and could not be changed. There was nothing she could do to help me, I'd tried everything and I didn't want her to call again. I also told her that I'd only agreed to see her under pressure from Dr. Sami and Frank. I didn't want her in my house. "You'd be wasting your time of you came back!" Poor woman!

Dr. D. eventually left, promising me (as if I cared!) that she would talk to her consultant about me (the one who told Frank I should get a job!!) to see if there was any drug other than Largactil, that could help me with the voices. She said she'd call again in a fortnight, even though I didn't want her to, as she couldn't come the following week because she was moving house!

Moving house? Brilliant CRAP!! That really made me feel like a whole lot more sh*tty rubbish! She couldn't come next week because moving house was more important than the risk of my

THE HUDDLE

children losing their mother! 'S**T! GET LOST!!!!! I knew I didn't want to see you!'.

Well of course moving house was more important to her than a suicidal patient! There are plenty of those about but you don't often move house! But she should never have let me cotton on to that! She should just have said she was coming again in a fortnight's time. Full stop. I was ill. I wasn't interested in her imminent house move. It was none of my business. I could not cope with this sort of personal information at the time it was given.

Dr. D. than glanced at our video collection and passed a jolly little comment,

"Oh! Your children watch the same sort of videos that my children watch!"

Wacko! I was TOTALLY thrilled. Yippee and wacky doo day!! I don't think! I didn't care a bloody damn, and didn't want to know anything like this! I was feeling very ill and my mind did not want to give room to anything other than my planned suicide. When? Where? How soon?

BUT! Fight it as I tried to, my mind could not let go of that tiny glimmer of hope that tried so hard to flicker in the dungeon of my mind. The hope that Dr. D would return with news of a cure-all-for-Janet drug. So I hung on. Somehow. Painfully. Miserably. I comforted myself with the knowledge that if she did not bring this good news for me, then that was the time to go.

Dr. D. came back. I was even polite enough to ask her how moving day went though I was not the slightest bit interested. Then she told me the news from her boss. There wasn't any more effective a drug than the Largactil I was already taking. I was devastated and sat there in stunned silence, trying to hold back the tears. Just as Dr. D. was about to leave,

"I don't want to see you again, there's no point!" The tears spilled over. I cried and talked but don't remember a thing I said. She eventually left with me insisting for the umpteenth time that I didn't want to see her or anybody else ever again. What was the point? They could offer me no cure. There was no miracle drug that could get rid of The Huddle. I think, even then, I already knew that deep down. Sometimes people clutch at any old straw, however ridiculous.

That was on a Thursday. I don't remember anything at all about the rest of that day or the long night that followed. Frank tells me that he dared not leave me at that time, and so I left him! He had popped across the road for only a few minutes to speak with a neighbour and, seeing my chance, I shot out of the house like a criminal escaping and ran up and over the hill and all the way to Dr. Sami's surgery which is not too far from where I live. I breathlessly asked for a prescription for sleeping tablets and (amazingly, incredibly, almost unbelievably!) I was handed one a few minutes later! That saved me having to buy Paracetamol, which I planned to do had the prescription for sleeping tablets been refused. I believed sleeping tablets would be quicker, and foolproof.

Five minutes later, I left the pharmacy clutching my box of pills, ran into the paper-shop next door to buy a can of coke to swill them down with, and began making my way to St. Woolos Cemetery. (We can see the cemetery from our back windows.)

THE HUDDLE

I was going to take my overdose there. I thought it was a good place to die – a cemetery!

However, just as I was waiting to cross the main road to the cemetery gates, my distraught husband, searching and running, caught up with me grabbed me roughly by the arm and pulled me home. Neither of us spoke a word. He flung me into a chair while he phoned the surgery to complain about the ease with which I'd been able to obtain a quantity of sleeping tablets, especially as Dr.Sami had warned him about keeping tablets away from me. (I would, however, point out that this prescription had not been signed by a doctor because I'd taken the same tablets before. It had been typed out on a computer by a receptionist and handed to me! Too easy!!!)

While Frank was on the phone, confused, desperate and upset, I sneaked quietly into the kitchen, managed to find some soluble Solpadol in the cupboard, and was in the process of dissolving them in water when I heard the phone click down and Frank came into the kitchen. Boy was he furious! (Looking back now, I can't say I blame him!!!)

"You really mean to do it, don't you?" Yes. I did. By way of reply I hurled the cup containing the fizzing Solpadol across the kitchen and repeatedly banged the sides of my head with my fists while I screamed and screamed. I'd finally lost it. Big time! I did not want to even *try* and stop myself. I didn't care a damn. Frank shook me and slapped me, whereupon I collapsed in a heap on the floor, still screaming. He carried me into the living-room and unceremoniously dumped me into a chair where I hugged and rocked myself, and carried on screaming and sobbing and wailing. I could not escape out of it all. The Huddle had won. They had finally driven me nuts and I didn't care a damn. I wanted to be dead more than I wanted anything else in the whole wide world and I embraced my evil comforter as my dearest, in fact my only, friend, my only comfort, the only one who understood how I felt.

When Frank did manage to get any words out of me, all I could gabble was that there were no tablets I could take, 'She said there weren't any..." there was nothing that could help me, nothing anyone could give me, nothing, nothing...

I spent the next couple of hours tearing my beloved collection of music books to shreds. All my piano music! Thirty years worth of collecting, hundreds of pounds worth of books, their sentimental value incalculable. Destroyed. Like I should have been. Frank sat and watched me do it and did absolutely nothing. All the times he had stopped me smashing dishes in the kitchen, but he didn't stop me destroying this amazing collection that I had once loved. Dishes could have been replaced. I cannot possibly hope to replace my music book collection. I am still devastated and heartbroken over my loss and cry often about it. Rightly or wrongly, I blame Dr. D. and I blame Frank. I should be blaming myself.

Pause. Make a cuppa. This is serious stuff.

Later….

THE HUDDLE

Anyway, where was I? Oh yes! Well, thankfully the kids had been in school while all the above was happening. Dr. Sami called to see me, summoned by one angry spouse, and following a quick call to St. Cadoc's I was given 200mg of Largactil and put to bed. I slept for four hours and was calm when I awoke. 'Bitch is awake!' A psychiatrist would be calling to see me that day, but never turned up. There was hardly any point! The one I'd seen the day before hadn't exactly helped matters! If anything, in the midst of the drug induced calmness, I was even more determined than ever to kill myself. I had already written all my suicide notes, plus a little book for my children to read when I was dead. Frank continued to stay with me, refusing Dr. Sami's offer to get me admitted to St. Cadoc's immediately.

"She will be safe there."
"No! I'll look after her myself at home."
"She must not be left!"
And I wasn't.   Damn it…………

What place has the recording of this episode in a chapter about drugs? Apart from anything else, it has been cathartic to write it all out and also illustrates that the only good I believed would come from drugs was if I took them as an overdose with the intention of ending my life. Tablets could only help me if they killed me. It's as simple as that.

The following Sunday night I had watched in stunned amazement and wonder as Jan went to work, acting as if everything was okay! Well, it was for her! It hadn't happened to her! She's just a bloody robot that goes to work!! Frank said that if he hadn't been absolutely sure that it was Jan going to work then he would not have dared let me out of the house. It was all so very weird, bizarre and unreal.

Another time when tablets, as an overdose, nearly helped me was at the beginning of September last year. It was a Monday, the day the kids had returned to school after the holidays and a day when Dr. Kapp was due to call. For some odd reason I was convinced that she would not turn up.

"She won't come! She won't come! Doesn't want to waste time on you, on you, on you, on you..."

August had been made just about bearable by the fact that the kids had been home although an attempt at a holiday away had proved disastrous. We had gone away on a Sunday and returned the very next day! I'd just not been well enough to cope. Neither was I well enough to cope with my children's return to school. I could not bear the thought of a day alone with The Huddle and Rachel etc. I'd reinforced my belief that the kids would be better off without me as their mother and the thought of Dr. Kapp not turning up left me feeling totally abandoned and desperate. An hour alone seemed too long. Seven hours alone until the kids came home did not, and could not, exist. I had planned for weeks what I would do on this day. So I did it!

I swallowed a lot of tablets.

"Go on, bitch! More, more, more, more, do it, do it, do it......"

A mixture of Paracetamol, sleeping tablets and Valium. I then put on my prettiest summer dress, a pearl necklace and my favourite red shoes. I

THE HUDDLE

arranged the bed tidily and lay down, ready to drift off to sleep and then die. I was very calm, and very hopeful that I would not fail. But I did. I didn't die. No more details here.

"Me want to write that in *my* book! Me write that bit, don't you, you don't know...."

That's Rachel, because the rest of that day is Rachel's story. It had been a terrifying day for her; and a disappointing one for me.

My poor, poor children.......

What were The Huddles' responses to my suicide attempts? Huh! – Boringly predictable! Great excitement! Absolute glee! Much encouragement! This further encourages my belief that they are external to me. If they were a part of me, then would they not have been accusing me of trying to kill them as well? Instead, they appeared to view my death as a relief from their own misery. Would my death mean freedom for them also? Freedom from having to exist as they do? Would they be transformed in some way? Or would they wander off in search of other food and end up tormenting somebody else?

The Huddle's reaction to my *failure* to kill myself was undisguised, utter contempt. I'd even failed at that, and they hated me for failing almost as much as I hated myself. I fail at living and I fail at death. I am not even able to kill myself. I am an utterly pathetic failure. Damn me. And damn them. Please!!

While I am writing about suicide I'd like to pick up on a few points from a conversation I was involved in a few days ago with our two close neighbours. They said this:

"I think that killing yourself, or even thinking about it, is the most wicked thing anyone could ever do."

"Yes, it's just *so* selfish!"

They didn't know about my suicidal thoughts and attempts, and as far as I knew, I was the only one of us who *had* thought about and attempted suicide. I had, and still have, this to say:

I am in many ways an extremely selfish person (Aren't we all at base level??). But, when I tried to kill me, selfishness did not come in to it. I really, really believed with all my heart that I would be doing everyone a favour by relieving them of the burden of me. My subsequent decision to live has, as far as I am concerned, been the most *unselfish* and the most pain filled decision I have ever made in the whole of my existence. Because it is not what I want. I am doing it for my children because I am told that they need me; I am not doing it for myself. I do not consider myself to be worth the enormous effort it takes to have to stay alive and *know* that I have to stay alive. Do I ever resent my children for keeping me alive? I'm ashamed to say that I sometimes do entertain such thoughts, but are they selfish? If I had never had children then I would not be here now and would not have inflicted life upon them, plus the misery of having a mother like me!

My poor, poor children.......

If Frank or one of my kids was depressed and suffering awful mental pain day in, day out, then I

THE HUDDLE

would not want them or expect them to make such a decision on *my* behalf! I know a little of what it's like for a mind to be in agony and I could not bear to see one of them suffering in this way and not knowing when, or even if, the pain would ever come to an end. I would cry over their pain but there would be tears of relief should they decide to end their pain by suicide. Sometimes it is the only pain relief available. If a patient in agony from a physical illness deliberately took an overdose of analgesia, then people would understand. There wouldn't be so much of a stigma attached to that sort of life ending. Who is it that truly understands the *mental* pain that leads to suicide? Who is it who can truly understand *my* pain at having to stay alive? I am told that suicide is wrong. Wrong for whom??????????????????

Enough! Let's get back to drugs! Anti-depressants!

"They won't f**king help you, you dull bitch…"

The most severe period of depression I have ever suffered began around this time two years ago and lasted, at the peak of its severity, for close to nine months. It was absolute agony, every second of every hour, day and night, week after week, and month after month. I felt dead. Isolated. Abandoned. Utterly without hope. Dr. Kapp would come. And she would go.

"I'll see you again in a month." She would tell me.

A month did not exist for me and each time she said that I knew that she would never again see me alive. When she did return four weeks later (because I *was* still alive) she was a complete stranger to me. Why was she bothering to come? Who was she? What was the point?

Frank and children did not exist. I did not speak to them. They were noisy shapes that moved about in front of my eyes. Rachel was terrified and clawed away at my skull, The Huddle were unbearable and Jan continued to ignore my state and go to work.

I was prescribed Lofepramine by Dr. Sami and Frank diligently fed them to me every day for about four weeks. I became worse and one evening was unable to stop crying. The dose of this antidepressant was increased. Still I continued to get worse, eventually abandoned the tablets altogether and refused to try an alternative. What was the point anyway? I didn't want to get better. I knew I wasn't going to get better. I wanted to die.

However, even without the help of drugs, I did eventually begin to emerge from this terrible darkness. Slowly. Painfully. I was reluctant to give up the devil I knew and face the fearful light that began to filter into my mind. Oh! The sheer terror of beginning to realise I was feeling better! How long would this feeling last? Was it for real? Dare I start to like it? Oh! And how closer to death I knew myself to be during those lightening days. September arrived, and the suicide attempt I have already described. I could not bear the thought of ever reaching that depth of misery again – better never to have seen the light??????????

Depression, in my experience, is a self limiting condition in that it will pass, but when? How does one begin to cope through those long, tortuous

THE HUDDLE

hours when drugs do not bring any relief and there is nothing whatsoever to cling to?

A characteristic of every period of depression I have ever suffered is the firm belief that, although you can acknowledge surviving previous depressions, this is the one you will *not* survive or recover from. Other depressions may have ended but this one is the father of all depressions, will never end and is therefore fatal. This one is utterly hopeless beyond all others and you will never feel any differently. There is absolutely no point or meaning to life. Life has no meaning, no value and no aim. You are a totally useless thing and suicide is the altruistic kindness that will rid the world of your burdensome, rotting existence.

I hate depression. I am terrified of it. I cannot escape it. It shadows me. It swallows me up, and then it retreats to lurk, waiting, ready for the next attack. Depression is cruel. It is a waste of time. It is a destroyer.

My drug situation at present is this: I do not take any prescribed medication regularly but I do take Largactil when I am wound up or desperate. I also take a sleeping tablet once or twice a week which enables me to get a guaranteed four hours sleep and at least manage seven or eight hours in bed. I might not be sleeping for all those hours, but I doze and my body has a rest. At the moment my insomnia is driving me nuts! How I wish that I could simply go to bed and sleep, but I cannot, however tired I may be. My mind is always too busy and will not be quiet and unhearing.

One thing I am trying, unsuccessfully, to do at the moment is give up taking too many painkillers.

Janet Cooper

I'm talking about four or five Paracetamol, or two Zydol, or three or four Nurofen Plus…… I take them because they relieve my almost constant headache, which at times is banging and nauseating. Too many can also make me drowsy, which is a 'pleasant' drowsiness compared to the lethargy induced by Largactil. When I am drug drowsy, my reception of The Huddle decreases – not as good as Largactil, but helpful enough to also allow me to potter about and get things done. I tried to explain to Dr. D. about the effects of a few too many painkillers in one dose but she was adamant that painkillers would not have this Huddle dulling effect on me. Ah well! She was the expert. I was only the idiot taking the damn things!! What did I know???........

I discovered the Huddle blurring effects of painkillers quite by accident. I had suffered agonies after having a tooth extracted due to an abscess and rang my dentist for advice. The tooth had been a little bugger to pull out, he wasn't surprised I was in a lot of pain, and advised me to try Nurofen Plus, which I did. Two did nothing for the pain. Three didn't either. Four really helped, also inducing the Huddle dulling drowsiness. (Honestly, Dr. D.! It really does happen this way for me!) And so began my analgesic habit.

I do realise that taking analgesia this way is not particularly good for me (although nobody has ever told me otherwise) but then that's just the way it has to be at present. I have to cope in whatever way I can. The Huddle are not particularly good for me either! Some people smoke, so instead of poisoning my lungs smoking I choose to poison my

THE HUDDLE

liver with painkillers. Which is worse? What the hell is the difference?

So. Medication. A brief chapter on. Not a good chapter but at least I've had a try.

"And f**king failed, you dull……"

They are in my desk lamp again. Looking at me. Laughing at me. And yes, they are right; it *is* a shame that there isn't a little white pill that will help me. I feel very bitter about that at times. As if the pharmaceutical companies have let me down!

In vain have I taken many medicines.
And they have not cured me.

CHAPTER NINE   CHRISTMAS 1996

"For unto you is born this day in the city of David a Saviour, which is Christ the Lord."   (Luke 2:3)

Do you remember Charles Dickens's masterpiece, 'A Christmas Carol', and what happened to the wonderful character, Scrooge? Well, I would like what happened to Scrooge to happen to me! No, no! I don't want to be visited at night by a trio of spooky spectres! But I do want to stop being a miserable, Christmas hating frump, and experience real joy and happiness this year. It would be such a change and it would make such a difference.

Wonderfully, amazingly this change has already begun to happen for me, but first of all let me tell you something about Charles Dickens. He was a voice hearer! I wanted you to know that. Frank claimed to have read this piece of information just before he met me and was astonished that Charles Dickens wrote so splendidly when he was obviously nuts. How on earth could a 'nutter' be clever, intelligent, and write books? Frank has since apologised to me for wrongly assuming that all people who hear voices are either complete nutters, Schizophrenics, or of low intelligence. I might not consider myself as particularly intelligent, but I am not schizophrenic and certainly not the style of 'nutter' Frank was referring to!

Another fascinating fact about Charles Dickens is that he was a Christian and passionately devoted to Christ. His last published work, which I have been reading this very morning (it's now 15th

THE HUDDLE

December 1996) is called "The Life of Our Lord" and was written expressly for his children. He never intended that it should be published. It tells the story of Jesus in simple language, suitable for a child, and is a most beautiful book to read. I wonder now if Mr. Dickens had to cope with blasphemous voices while he wrote it. I wonder how his voices affected him. How *did* he cope with them? Interesting.

So far, three people have been instrumental in changing Christmas for me this year. They are Sir Edward Heath, my neighbour, Kath, and Dr. Kapp, in that order. So let me explain Sir Edward's part in my transformation first.

(FIDDLESTICKS!!! That is my euphemism for 'Oh S**t!' I cannot write this chapter. Rip the damn thing up. Rip it all up. What is the point. Can't write this. Damn it!!

Minutes and hours and days and weeks go past. Somehow.

The Christmas I was writing about has now come and gone, but I'll return to the account of it, because if I don't, then The Huddle will have scored a victory and I don't want that to happen. Boring, boring drivel it might well be, but I've got this far – I'm going to finish this book! Huddle, worms, whatever..... So let's get back to Sir Edward.)

It was the end of November, and a bitterly cold and wet day. Jan had worked a night shift, the kids had left for school and hubby was in work. I was cold, miserable and overtired when the letterbox rattled and there on the mat lay a parcel from the House of Commons. What the...? I double and triple checked that it was really, really addressed to me before gingerly opening it. Inside was a brand new Carol book sent by Sir Edward Heath!

Remember all those music books I'd destroyed? One of them had been a most favourite book of carols compiled by Sir Edward that I'd loved and used for many years. With Christmas fast approaching I'd begun to miss it so much! Frank had tried in vain to find a replacement copy for me and had, in desperation, written to Sir Edward to ask if the book was still being published and by whom. Instead of simply sending this information, Sir Edward had so kindly sent me a copy of the book together with a letter expressing his good wishes for the coming Christmas time. I was stunned and thrilled and sat on the settee hugging that special book and crying my eyes out. I held my breath as I looked through its pages, the words, music and pictures so familiar to me that it was like the return of some faithful friend!

I wrote back to Sir Edward, thanking him, and explaining a little about how much his gift had meant to me; it was like a light being turned on for Christmas and I was absolutely delighted.

A week later a letter arrived from the House of Commons to tell me that Sir Edward had received my thanks and was glad I was so pleased with the book. Pleased? That was a bit of an understatement! I was over the moon!! And began to happily and enthusiastically play the beautiful carols and songs that it contained. Had Sir Edward

THE HUDDLE

not sent me this book, then I doubt if *any* Christmas music would have been played on my piano that particular festive season.

This kind gift had a bit of a knock on effect too. Rachel gingerly peeped out of her awful depression one afternoon while I was sat at the piano.

"Me play? Please?"

"Okay then."

Next thing I know, she's playing a carol and teaching Katy to sing the words. It was weird, but very beautiful and moving and we all ended up crying – but good tears this time! I remember Rachel saying that she ought to play this carol for Elinor (Dr. Kapp) just to show her that witches can change side and sing to Jesus like angels! I think that Dr. Kapp, Elinor, knows that a 'witch' can change sides as she still watches us struggling with that change.

"You can't get out of it, witch bitch, come back, come join us, come back, Satan's little bittle puppet....."

"Hark the herald angels sing,".... We sing aloud to drown The Huddle out, and just for a moment there is something or Someone so lovely inside me, us, that it is overwhelming. Like God is in our head......

Thank-you Sir Edward!

Then came the afternoon of Sunday December 1st.

"Come down for a cuppa!" Invited our neighbours. I am not allowed to go into other folks' homes, I find it exceedingly difficult, but we accepted their invitation and I was later to be very glad that we did.

Now Kath is a little older than me, with a pretty, gentle face, and has never had children. Nevertheless, she displayed a wonderfully childlike and infectious joy and excitement over the season of Christmas. Her tree lay on the living-room carpet waiting to be put upright and decorated, and a little tree in the garden had already been adorned with glittery balls. Kath told me that she could hardly wait for the 1st December because this was the day, every year, without fail, when she put up her tree and trimmings. Her face glowed with pleasure and I was caught up in her joy and infected with her innocent delight and enthusiasm.

I was, in fact, so impressed that our humble Christmas decorations were lovingly and enjoyably dug out of the attic and arranged around our home that very same day! The Huddle were horrified! I was pleased. I was definitely feeling a bit friendlier towards Christmas.

Thanks Kath!

Then came the first Yuletide torment in earnest. I found that I could not sit in my usual chair because it was right next to the Christmas tree. The Huddle had filled the tree and my chair with the beetles which usually only live in my pillow. The branches of the Christmas tree became huge and menacing, pretty baubles clanged against each other like the bells of hell, and the tinsel that had been draped over pictures around the room squirmed into life as hissing serpents.

THE HUDDLE

I fought it. I coped with it. I hated it. At times I wanted to become wild and uncontrolled, hurling the Christmas tree out of existence. I did quite well though, and lasted until Boxing Day, when the kids showed their disappointment and wondered why the decorations were put away so early. They had to go as I don't think I could have coped with them for much longer. My poor, poor children….

Dr. Kapp had visited again on the 16th and further encouraged me in my efforts to enjoy Christmas. As she pointed out, I was free to choose what to do. I could either give in to the Huddle and have the usual thoroughly miserable time, or else I could put up with The Huddle's sabotage attempts but at the same time make a supreme effort to enjoy Christmas. Either way, The Huddle were out to torment me and have a field day over the Christian festival. Therefore, if they were going to go 'over the top' anyway, whatever I did, then I really *did* have a choice! Enjoy it and they'd torment me. Hate it and they'd torment me. So I chose to enjoy it.

Thanks Dr. Kapp! Not bad for a shrink!

All went quite well until the early hours of Christmas morning, although I suppose it all began to go pear shaped exactly a week before Christmas day, on the 18th December.

Jan had arrived home from work aching all over and with a sore, tight, chest, and we spent the next two days in bed feeling too ill and feverish to get up. I had caught a nasty cold from Frank and son, Frank's cough being even louder than his booming sergeant major voice and jolting my throbbing head at every paroxysm! Added to the miseries of the common coryza (although mine felt decidedly *un*common!) I was experiencing the worst period pains I'd had for years and had also developed a mouth full of painful ulcers. Wonderful! All right before Christmas!

Now I'd read in one of the gossipy women's magazines that ones (*ones????)* immune system can become considerably lowered due to the stresses and strains of this time of year, thus making one (one?) more susceptible to infections. So be it. That was me then. I had feared that I'd subconsciously set out to be ill as a way of opting out of Christmas. But that was daft! After all, I didn't choose to catch the damn cold, did I! It was only my daughter who didn't succumb to this wretched bug, and for nearly a week the house was filled with the sound of coughing and the smell of Vick.

On the day before Christmas Eve I was feeling better. We all were. The kids had gone to bed, The Huddle were in the television, Christmas music was floating around and I was playing Scrabble with Frank. (I was winning as usual!)

"Turn that f**king holy crap off! TURN THAT OFF! TURN THAT OFF! TURN THAT…"

I made a concentrated effort to listen to the music The Huddle were telling me to turn off. It was a recording of Josef Locke singing 'Adeste Fideles' with that incredible voice of his, and it was the most beautiful, haunting rendition of this lovely carol that I had ever heard. Bliss! I was entranced and yet filled with pain. Contrary to the words he sung, his voice conveyed to me the tragic tones of somebody

THE HUDDLE

who was alone in the world, and indeed this alcoholic who died in the gutter no doubt experienced this utter loneliness. I was reminded of 'The voice of one crying in the wilderness, prepare ye the way of the Lord.' (Matthew 3:3) and yet he was singing 'Adeste Fideles', O come all ye faithful. I suppose it does go together is some way, does it not? As I continued to listen, still, unmoving, and completely taken up with the music and singing, I was filled with beauty and an exquisite agony.

Christmas Eve arrived and was a busy, happy day with me managing to keep going and remain tolerably tuned out of The Huddle. Then during the evening I stirred my coffee twenty eight times and burst into tears.

"What's the matter love?" asked Frank.

I told him.

"Well, take seven stirs off then."

"How do I do that?" I asked, puzzled.

"Seven *anti*clockwise stirs, which leaves you with twenty one clockwise stirs." He answered, logically. So that's what I did, and it worked, but I was left decidedly unsettled.

We all went to bed at the same time and two excited kids finally fell asleep. I couldn't sleep and lay awake into the early hours of Christmas morning, unable to tune out of The Huddle much, but too dog tired and fed up to go downstairs. Hodie Christus natus est! Christ is born today! – And The Huddle wanted to strangle this infant at birth. Et cetera. I won't write it down. I lay there struggling against the noisy sobs which would have woken Frank. I felt as if a huge black shutter had come thumping down inside my mind and I became aware of Rachel crying silently and pitifully, her hands wrapped around her head. Janny, little Janny, was making her sad little noises.

What this sudden shutter had done was to cut me off from all the season's excitement, joy, tinsel, Christmas trees, baubles, gifts, toys, busy shops, carol singers, fairy lights, happy kids, pretty cards, festive food and a Merry Christmas one and all! It was all suddenly gone and everything was bare and raw and lonely. All that was left was the memory of the birth of a baby called Jesus, and that did not fill me with joy. In fact I was in agony over it. "Fear and the pit and the snare are upon thee, O inhabitant of the earth." (Isaiah 24:17) The birth of Jesus frightens me the same as it frightens The Huddle, for all their arrogant, blasphemous ranting and raving. His birth. This is the struggle, the battle, the fury of Satan and the whole of hell against the coming of a Saviour, Jesus Christ. "...the Son of God was manifested that he might destroy the works of the devil." (1 John 3:8) Reverend H preached a sermon on that verse at a carol service I attended shortly after he diagnosed me as possessed. I was afterwards taken to the Manse and exorcised. Oh! Miserable Christmas that was! It made the voices ten times worse.

Anyway. Why then does Jesus *not* destroy the works of the devil, if that's what He came to do? Hatred, abuse, sin and death and destruction, disease, poverty, Satan, all manner of evil and wickedness, the spiritual servants of hell, The Huddle... Jesus was born to die and we are told that he triumphed on the cross for each one of us. Who, then, is sharing in that triumph? Is Father

THE HUDDLE

God holding back the power and the evidence of this triumph? Shall we only truly experience it in heaven? That is, after we die? What, then, is the point of life? It is the secret mystery of God! We are allowed no secrets from Him, and yet……

The birth of a Saviour and the fury of hell, as represented by The Huddle, all mixed up and battling away inside us. Me. And I was in agony. The Huddle laughed at me and there was no way to be comforted. "Long is the way, and hard that leads up to the light." (John Milton, Paradise Lost)

Thankfully that Christmas Eve night came to an early end when the kids bounced onto the bed at just after four o'clock. (Four o'clock??? Yep! Bloomin' four o'clock!!!) I managed to smile and attempted to enjoy all the excitement and rush of opening presents and stockings. My children had bought me four cast iron door wedges, so I knew I must stay alive and wait for good weather so that I could wedge a few doors open. Inside Rachel was acting devastated at not receiving one card or present. But she never does! It's awkward! How many people know her for goodness sake? I cannot buy her anything because she would not take anything from me. Frank sent her a card last year with angels on it, but nothing this year, even though she speaks to him nearly every day. I can almost say 'poor Rachel', but then she knows the difficulty of the situation. It isn't easy. Am I supposed to buy presents for all of us? Buy for one and do the rest get jealous? Awkward.

I wonder what Siamese twins do on their birthdays and at Christmas. Do they buy each other gifts? How on earth would they keep it as a surprise until the day? It's all very weird and bizarre.

I cannot write this chapter.

Yes. I can!

Rachel has accused my husband of not buying her a Christmas present. But he did!
"Me write?" (That's her!)
"You write then." (That's me!) This is what Rachel wrote –

' Janet says it's Friday 3rd January 1997 (6.25p.m.) and I just said to Frankie that he didn't buy me a Christmas present and I had been very upset so he said that he did and took me upstairs and got a little present out of the wardrobe. It is like a glass ball with an angel in it and when you shake it, it snows. I like it and it is mine. I have never ever had a Christmas present before and it makes me want to start crying. This is almost my best writing but it doesn't matter and I don't know what the others think about me getting a present and they not getting one. I don't see why I should not have something. Jesus had presents. Janet did not have much for Christmas. Go now. I go now.'

This is what Jan wrote –

'Jan. Mother hen Jan. I am not obviously present when I am (infrequently) here, but I am aware of what is going on. I suddenly feel I could write many pages, but hold back, knowing that

THE HUDDLE

Janet will read this. Liz and Katy can write their own comments on how they feel about Christmas. Liz write. Come on.'

This is what Liz reluctantly wrote –

'Don't want to. Do not <u>care</u> about anything and <u>hate</u> everybody and you are all <u>nasty</u> very <u>nasty</u>. Go away. Me go back now. Liz.'

'Go back now. Katy write a sentence. Katy write now.' (Jan)

'I do not think that Christmas is for me.
                By Katy.'

'Janny is too young to write. She accepts how things are. Two others must not exist. Rachel wants to finish this page. Rachel' – (Jan)

'I did not <u>want</u> to write about this in Janet's book. Wanted it for <u>my</u> book. But I don't care. Sign your name. Why? Sign my name.
                Rachel. S**t

Where was I? Oh yes! Christmas Eve night. And yes, I do know what has just been written although I do not remember it coming about. I wish the elusive Jan had written more and given more information. If she is reading this then maybe she will take the hint and write or type more. Please? I want to know.

Right. Back to Christmas Eve night! I had not had a 'silent night, holy night, all is calm, all is bright'. It had been more like 'Herod the King, in his raging....', taking Herod to be symbolic of hell's fury at Christ's incarnation. Jesus born to die. How tragic. 'Then of the thorns they made a crown, and with rough fingers pressed it down, till on His forehead fair and young, red drops of blood like roses sprung.' Exquisite agony!

Can't write this chapter.

"She can't write this chapter! You dull, fat useless......"

Yes I can! And will!!!

Imaginary reader! (You still with us?) Think about this. If you were to be denied all the commercial trappings of Christmas, all the hype, gifts, gathering of family and friends, time off work etc., and there was nothing at all left to you but the knowledge of the birth of Christ, how would you feel? Relieved about not having to shop, spend money, cater for others, and appear to be enjoying it all? Or would there be just nothing, like any other month of the year? Would you expect and hope to experience joy over the remembrance of a Divine birth? Would this memory be enough for you if

THE HUDDLE

nothing else went with it? Do you think much about Christ's birth at this time of year? If so, what does it mean to you? Joy? Gratitude? Wonder? Unbelief? Or, as it means for me, pain? What is wrong with me that I should feel like this? Always, always, always I am so very sorry for the way I am.

Throughout Christmas Day and Boxing Day my efforts at dissimulation crumbled under the constant onslaught of The Huddle plus Rachel's angry, hurt sulkiness.

"I was not sulking!" (That's her now.)

"Yes you were. Because you didn't have a present the same time as the rest of us!" (That's me.)

"Was <u>not</u> sulking!!"

"Oh for goodness sake…"

"SHUT-UP! And leave me <u>ALONE!!!</u>"

I became very depressed and due to this, plus the after effects of the bad cold, I spent two days curled up in a chair, eyes shut, feeling incredibly sleepy and barely able to open my eyes for long. I was aware of what was going on, of my kids playing happily, of being at my mother's for Christmas dinner, but I did not feel a part of it all. As everyone tucked in to a feast of a dinner, I spread jam thinly onto two slices of toast, even then not managing to eat all of it. I wondered how many other people felt empty after Christmas dinner. Sad!

Whilst curled up in my solitude, yet never alone, The Huddle bombarded me with all the bad memories of Christmases past that I had fully intended giving thought room to prior to Christmas Day in order to package them up and throw them away. I hadn't got round to it, coward that I am, afraid of the memories, the feelings and the tears. I am so afraid of crying. Won't think about them or write about them even now. I am not a brave person. So many Christmases with The Huddle. Why am I not strong enough to overcome them? Why am I so weak, selfish and self pitying?

Now Christmas is all over. The year is new and I am filled with dread. Another year to be got through? How? Will somebody please tell me how? And why? What am I supposed to do? Angel (Dr.Kapp?) now gently reminds me,

"Just get through today. That's all."

Sensible advice that can work, but then she will no doubt say the same thing tomorrow, and the next day, and the day after that. How I *want* to wish that the incontrovertible truth was that I shall not be here for another Christmas. How wonderful it would be to hang on to that comfort, but I cannot. The evil comforter is gone and by making my decision to live I must struggle on with it. Whatever. I should rather be wishing that I shall never have another Christmas like the one that has just come and gone! Can it get better? Can it get worse? How can I face another year with The Huddle? I don't want to, so how, then, do I get rid of them? Is it ever a possibility? WHAT THE HELL AM I GOING TO DO???? Jesus says, deep inside my head, "Trust Me!"

Lord I believe, help thou mine unbelief.......

The Huddle are now in my desk lamp. It is a different lamp since Christmas but they don't mind

THE HUDDLE

that, as long as they are close enough to my typing. Angel reminds me not to be frightened by the worms. How can I not be frightened by worms squirming through my typewriter keys? Has she sprayed them with some Divine wormicide? Angel dust to get rid of the nasties?

Lord, sprinkle them with heavenly dust my mind, the butterfly, the desk lamp, Tesco's stamp machines, the bars of soap in the bathroom, the kettle .... please? Do not make me be of this world, but take us close to Thee, and give silence. Please give us a quiet head. God be in our head! And silence.

Oh! Still the jarring sounds of earth
That round the pathway ring,
And bid the toilers rest awhile
To hear the angels sing.   AMEN.

CHAPTER TEN   THE HUDDLE AND MARRIED LIFE

"...a man... shall be joined unto his wife, and they two shall be one flesh." (Ephesians 5:31)

My husband is convinced beyond a shadow of a doubt that he has been blessed with the most wonderful male appendage in the whole wide world. I should have realised on our very first date (he took me to see 'Confessions of a window cleaner', followed by an *attempted* grope in a dingy bedroom) that he was insatiably addicted to satisfying this little animal that lurks inside his Mickey Mouse boxer shorts. As I write this, I realise that he will balk at the word 'little' when applied to Willy the Wonderful! Yet after listening to much gross exaggeration I am relieved to report that this most magnificent, unique creature is not twelve inches long, six inches in circumference and hewn out of granite. As far as I'm concerned, unexcited male appendages resemble nothing more than the scrawny necks of plucked chickens, just hanging around - rejects from the cat food factory. They are not a pretty sight!

I am being silly. I know. It is my vain attempt to cover my embarrassment and reluctance to write such a chapter. Why bother if I find it awkward? Because I believe it will help me to think a few things through, and writing is a good way for me to do that. How do I begin? Probably by jumping right in at the deep end and admitting that having sex with the Huddle around is a misery. And that's an understatement!!

THE HUDDLE

I will always try to reject any counselling or therapy that attempts to deal with my sex life because I like to pretend I don't have one! But what counselling I *have* received has informed me that sex is not dirty, sinful, satanic or only for the conception of children. However, knowing all this intellectually, that is, with my mind, does not mean that I believe or feel in with my heart, and I will still avoid sex as much as possible. Dr. Kapp points out that I am a married woman, sex is a normal part of that relationship, my husband has needs and it is unfair of me to try and deny him totally. So we arrive at the conclusion that my husband needs sex, but I don't. My husband wants sex, but I don't. My husband enjoys sex, but I don't. My husband thinks there is nothing wrong with sex, but I think that there's *everything* wrong with it!!

So Dr. Kapp then encouraged me to change my whole attitude to the whole subject, deal with my bad feelings and memories, then, if all that fails, to view sex as a gift I am able to give my husband in order to give him this pleasure.

WHAT??? BOLLOCKS TO ALL THAT! LITERALLY!!!

Why should *I* have to be totally unselfish and struggle through agonies trying to make sex okay for me so that my husband can have a few seconds of ecstasy once or twice a week? Why can't *he* be encouraged to be the totally unselfish partner and go through a few 'agonies' to get used to *not* having sex with me? (There is a lock on the bathroom door, you know!) Why has it got to be *me* fighting all the damn battles? I have the misery of living because I know my children need a mother. Now I'm to have the misery of putting up with sex for my husband! What about ME???

"Self pitying little bitch she is …. See fat, dirty…."

Yes. I am self pitying and dirty. I feel filthy, rotten dirty, especially after sex when it is impossible to get clean. Ah! I hear you saying that there is still really no argument as sex is a normal and expected part of married life. Well, my answer to that is a resounding NO **IT DAMN WELL ISN'T!!!!** Sex for me is not normal in any way. How can it be? I have The Huddle. I have Rachel and the others. I have been raped. I have dabbled in the occult. I have been given advice by the rather quaint, keep-it under-the-bedclothes-with-the-light-off, unqualified-to-give-such-advice Reverend H and his spouse. Sex never was, is not, and never can be normal for me.

It might be easier for me to deal with my difficulties under the five categories I've just mentioned. The Huddle. Multiple Personality. Rape. Occultism. Reverend H. Each title, as you will soon discover, imaginary reader, brings its own problems. Mix them all together to make me, and then it is a recipe for disaster when it comes to any attempt at a sexual relationship with my husband. I shall deal with the Huddle last of all because they won't like that – being the last to get attention on this subject.

THE HUDDLE

Multiple personality. I live with Jan, Rachel, Liz, Katy and Janny. We share the same body. So if I hate having sex, couldn't one of the others have it for me? Instead of me? Then all I might be left with is the washing and trying to get clean afterwards but without any actual memory of the act of intercourse. This indeed is the way it was until quite recently. I would deliberately refuse to be present and, as far as I know, it was Rachel having sex with my husband. She is only seventeen but I didn't seem to care, as long as it didn't have to happen to me. My husband was aware of what was going on, but as I would become absent only *after* the start of his amorous advances, there was very little he could be expected to do about it. So he says. Dr. Kapp more or less backed this up by telling me that men reach a point of 'no return', so it must have been very difficult for him. (Poor love!) It wasn't exactly a doddle for me, either! It was also profoundly disturbing for Rachel who has spent the last two years willingly converting herself from being a slut, a demon and a witch into a chaste and modest Christian.

So Rachel began doing the same as I had been doing; becoming absent during sex and pushing forward either Liz or Katy. Thankfully it didn't get as far as little Janny! All this got me out of having sex alright, but at a price. It was often difficult to be 'me' again afterwards and my husband would spend hours trying to calm us all down and get me back in control of this body again. I would be confused, distressed and agitated. The others began cutting me more and were becoming seriously disturbed and traumatised by what was happening to them.

(So why didn't my husband back off??? If he found sex so difficult, I would never, ever do it with him!)

Dr. Kapp stepped into the situation (not literally!!) and pointed out that it was unfair and even cruel of me to push the others into an adult sexual situation, considering their ages and the fact that they are already very damaged and hurt personalities. She said I'd have to stop doing it and begin having sex with my husband myself, however difficult, seeing that I was the one that was married to him. I did listen carefully to what Dr. Kapp was saying and knew on some level that she was right. Damn it!

I began making the effort to stay 'me' during sex. It was and is horrible. I don't like it and it's not what I want. I was, and still am, frequently aware of the terror of the others in case I should again out one of them in my place, and I now realise a little of the misery I was putting them through. Rachel does not want to see, hear, or have any knowledge of this part of my marriage, and yet at one time she...... She curls up in her cell with her hands clapped tight over her ears and her eyes tight shut.

I managed to stick being 'me' for several months but then realised I was becoming absent again during sex. According to Rachel it was nothing to do with her, Liz or Katy, and my husband assured me it was definitely me! But I knew that it definitely wasn't!! Could it be Jan? Are we sort of partly integrated without me knowing about it? Or do I hate having sex so much that I have developed the ability to indulge in a little selective amnesia?

So that's how it is. My body is used for sex, but I'm not always certain who my husband's partner is.

THE HUDDLE

He may speak afterwards about what has taken place and I'll not know what he's on about. I might even deny that what he says took place, did actually take place.

"No, that's not possible. I wouldn't have done that …… wouldn't have said that…. That's not me!"

Most alarming of all is when hubby claims that 'I' have enjoyed sex! Maybe he's trying to convince *himself* of that! For me, to enjoy sex would be to condone rape. I will never enjoy it. It is not allowed. No go!!

I've just had a thought. I wonder what God thinks about all this? (God has a multiple personality. Father, Son and Holy Spirit. So has the sun. Light, heat and radiation.) Is my husband guilty of adultery if he knowingly has sex with one of the others? Is he guilty of repeated rape because none of us consent to sex? Am I guilty of forcing two teenagers and a twelve year old into having sex? Would God judge Frank and I on these matters? Or would that only be the judgement of the Reverend H's harsh, punishing, literal God? When my husband married me, did he marry by body regardless of who is obviously present in it at any one time and is therefore entitled to have sex with whomever? What *is* God's view of it all? Is He angry with me for the way that I am, we are?

Maybe God Himself becomes absent and sends Jesus instead, who will envelope the whole confusing situation with His infinite patience and understanding, his forgiveness as necessary, and His unconditional love to us all as we seek to find a way of coping with an extremely awkward situation. O Lord, please, be kind and gentle with each one of us. Be understanding. "Marriage is honourable in all, and the bed undefiled." (Hebrews 13:4) If only it felt that way……

Gee I hate sex! Let's change the subject for a while shall we? Today is Friday 10th January 1997 and something unusual happened this morning. I went to the hairdresser. That in itself is not unusual because I keep my hair cropped very short – another form of cutting – but what happened *while* I was there is what's unusual. It might not seem like much to you but it really distressed me and caused a lot of unease. The Huddle jumped into the hairdryer that was hanging on a hook underneath the mirror in front of which I was sitting, and they have never, ever done that before.

Unless I am in a different place for longer than about thirty minutes (my wet cut takes no more than twenty) then The Huddle will not go to the bother of inhabiting an object, preferring to remain around my head. Today, however, they were obviously intent on unnerving me and they unfortunately succeeded because I sat there in sheer terror of the hairdresser drying me off with this Huddle infested hairdryer. I didn't want them blown at my head, to cling to me and claw away at my skull. I did not want them hurled furiously at me in a blast of hot air, coming at me, blown at my head, coming at me, coming at me, coming at me….

As the hairdresser finished snipping away and went to grasp this dryer, I jumped in quickly and politely refused to be 'dried off', pointing out that as my hair was so very short it would dry on its own in

THE HUDDLE

no time at all. The girl shrugged her shoulders, quite happy, and probably thought nothing more of it. The Huddle were furious and I felt that I'd managed to outwit them as they'd mocked and cackled away from the little dryer.

Going to the hairdresser is not, for me, the treat many women find it to be. It is simply a means to an end. I very rarely gaze at myself in a mirror because I see others looking out at me, I am afraid of suddenly seeing The Huddle surrounding my head, and I am not a pretty sight anyway! To have my hair cut, I am sat in front of a large, well lit mirror, trying at all times to avoid eye contact with Rachel who always keeps a watchful eye on the proceedings.

"She's not going to stick those scissors in my eyes, is she?"

"No." I reply. "Of course she isn't!" Isn't she?

"Just look at her….look at yourself, you ugly f**king cow you! She getting cut, cut, cut, cut, cut, cut, cut slut, cut slut, snip and kill and snip and kill and snip and kill…….."

After washing my hair with semi congealed blood, the stylist snipped away and wet hair stuck to me in little dark clumps like brooding insects. Worms slithered down the neck of my blouse, making me itchy and squirmy, and at any moment my head could have been gashed open. Strange hands moved quickly about my head, wielding a lethal instrument.

"She gonna cut your FRIGGING head OFF!!! Fat ugly...."

Other women in various, ridiculous stages of torment littered the room as we sat there, hating it, and wanting to get out as quickly as possible.

As I escaped the chamber of horror I gasped, emerging as I did into a bitterly cold winter's day with very damp hair. Damn and blast The Huddle! They caught up with me, settling back into the space around my head as I made my way home. They kept telling me that I looked dreadful, bald, even uglier, like a freak, and everyone was looking at me and laughing at us. Damn them to hell!!

Now The Huddle are in the butterfly. They are trying to puzzle me and keep my attention today, as they are usually in the desk lamp when I type. So why have they now decided to be different? Why?

While we are on the subject of hair, I've just remembered that Reverend H used to accuse me of worshipping my long, auburn tresses. "...if a woman has long hair, it is a glory to her..." (1 Corinthians 11:15) Well, Mr. Crackers Reverend! – Rest assured that I am now well and truly stripped of my glory! I no longer have it because when I was anorexic I shaved the beautiful stuff off and wore a scarf to hide my baldness and my shame. Totally stripped of any glory, I have kept it boyishly short ever since. Satisfied Mr. Reverend? And, Mr. Reverend, while we are on the subject of 'cutting' – I had never, ever cut myself enough to need suturing until you started to deal with me! Pin pricks, scrapes and deep scratches there were plenty of, but no deep, gaping gashes pouring with

THE HUDDLE

blood, week after week, requiring many stitches. You, Sir, did not do me much good!

And ah! What sad thought! If Jesus were to come to me this very minute, I would wash his feet with my tears, but I could not now gently wipe them dry with my hair. I have *no* beauty now, save Him. Maybe that's a good thing!

I have digressed somewhat. So what! This is supposed to be a book for getting things off my chest.

Right! What's the next put-me-off-sex category that I'll deal with?
Rape! That's the one, so let's just go for it eh?

RAPE! Even the word sounds evil and is difficult and brutal to pronounce. Rape is the forced, painful piercing of the body and the total destruction of the spirit. When it happens at an early age and steals the flower of sweet innocence, the mind defends itself by creating another person for it to happen to. Then you can stare at nothing and not be there.

Rape is the shattering of childhood innocence, it robs a husband of legitimate intimacy and secret knowledge of his wife, it is utterly humiliating and a total violation of privacy. Rape produces an ejaculation of the slimy and everlasting entrails of dirtiness, self loathing, guilt and zero self esteem. Rape is a crime. It is wrong, evil, wicked, and NOT the fault of the victim, but try telling the victim that! I have been raped. I'm not going into any more details – just those four words. I have been raped.

Having sexual intercourse reminds me of being raped. That is the difficulty, simply put. My mind and The Huddle will play tricks on me and I will feel that again and again and again I am being raped and re-raped and re-raped. The flashbacks are terrible. Sudden. Loud. Vivid. Glorious technicolour. I will feel, see and smell everything to do with rape. I will feel a rapist inside me, smell him, gasp under his forced weight, try to push him off and be back in the same location. Flash, flash, flash. I will cry bitter tears, I will not be me, I will hold my head in my hands and feel nothing but the pain of remembering. I will remember physical pain, between my legs, my arms roughly handled, a kick to my right thigh and the bang of my head on the floor. Then came the soreness and the bleeding and the terrible, terrible secrecy.

My mind bled with secrets long before my arms and my body did. Somebody once told me to 'put all that behind you – it's all in the past', but they couldn't tell me *how* to put it all behind me!! (This person had never been raped by the way!) It isn't all in the past! Rape is relived week after week after week, and never leaves me. It's not that I *want* to remember and have all these flashbacks. I don't! But I cannot stop them happening. I've tried!!!

Feel like another little gem from Reverend H? Wait for it – this is a prize one! It's so unbelievable I'll put it in capital letters and underline it!

<u>I WAS MADE TO PRAY FOR FORGIVENESS FOR MY PART, HOWEVER SMALL, IN BEING RAPED!</u>

"There *must* have been a part of you that went along with it Janet!"

NO! NO!! NO!!! NO!!!!!!!!!!

THE HUDDLE

There was no part of me that went along with it! NO! A thousand times NO!!! The Reverend was cruelly ignorant on this subject!

I don't want to type any more words about rape. It's starting to upset me and I'm kooky enough as it is! I'm sure you're intelligent enough to see how the experience of being raped impacted seriously on the intimate side of my marriage, No more on this now. Change the subject then. Okay. Will do.

A bit of silliness! Do you know what a Babushkaphobic is? Babushkaphobia is an aversion to one's own grandchildren! How awful! How about an Autochondriac? This refers to somebody morbidly concerned with the well being of their car. They are forever washing and polishing the damn thing and checking the bodywork for dents and scratches. They frequently imagine they can hear the sounds of mechanical failure. Fascinating eh? One last bit of silliness – when my husband told me ages ago that another name for diarrhoea was the Aztec two-step I howled with laughter! On now with the subject of this chapter….

Sex and the occult. "Rebellion is as the sin of witchcraft." (1 Samuel 15:23) And sure enough, in the practice of witchcraft and Satanism the idea is to rebel as much as possible against the laws of God as set down in scripture and whether or not you *know* you are rebelling against God doesn't bother the devil at all! For example, there's the upside down cross, the devil's 666, the satanic version of the Christian communion service et cetera. Sexually, this gives freedom to carry out all manner of fornication, obscene acts and exhibitionism. The more explicit and perverted the better, as far as this prince of darkness is concerned. Anything goes.

When 'hyped up' within the confines of a group, meeting, coven – sex can be extremely intense and exquisitely pleasurable, the drive is on and on and on to an abnormal orgasmic frenzy. But you don't even need to be with others for this to happen. Alone and open to the world of the demonic, they require no persuasion to use you for the purpose of sexual gratification, whether you are willing or not. If you are not willing then it's a case of demonic rape. How utterly humiliating! So what exactly am I implying here? Sex with a demon? Is it possible to have sex with, for example, one of The Huddle? Spiritually, yes it is, and pleasure, though unwanted, can be intensely physical, or else it can mean the pain and violation of rape. Ask Rachel!

"Leave me alone! I don't do that any more! I don't!"

But "be not deceived: neither fornicators, nor idolators, nor adulterers… shall inherit the Kingdom of God." (1 Corinthians 9&10)
Gaining sexual pleasure from the spirit world would have made us all three! A fornicator. An idolator. An adulterer. Not very nice, but then, "And such were some of you: but ye are washed, ye are sanctified, but ye are justified in the name of the Lord Jesus, and by the Spirit of our God." (1 Corinthians 6:11)

So I know that God has forgiven us my wicked and evil occult practices and all that they involved.

THE HUDDLE

The problem is that I do not *feel* forgiven and I most certainly do not feel clean and pure in the sight of God! "Me does a bit!" Rachel does a bit. Possibly because she no longer has sex? "Now the body is not for fornication but for the Lord." (1 Corinthians 6:13) "Flee fornication ... know ye not that your body is the temple of the Holy Ghost?" (1Corinthians 6:18&19)

Worshipping Satan is opposite to worshipping God. I don't believe there is any greater opposite. Therefore changing sides brings many difficulties both spiritually and emotionally, not least of all where sex is concerned. I had been led and encouraged to think that to enjoy sex was to glorify and please the devil. Hence sexual pleasure reminds me of Satan, hence my decision to never enjoy it. And if the devil wants you to go overboard and have a whale of a time, does God expect the opposite?

Reverend H, when I was in the very early stages of wanting to become a Christian, told me, concerning sex, that I should have some sense of 'need', and then went on to rebuke me strongly when I foolishly told him I had once, long ago, woken Frank in the middle of the night seeking to satisfy this 'need'!

"You do *not* wake your husband in the middle of the night simply because you have an urge, Janet!"

May I add that what my husband raised was certainly not an objection! Mrs. Reverend also suggested that I would feel safer having sex underneath the bedclothes, at night time and with the light off. Apparently the middle of the afternoon when the kids weren't around was *not* an appropriate time to get together! Another of her suggestions was that I should pray during sex that it would be over as quickly as possible. All this, and more, gave me the impression that sex within the Christian faith wasn't *quite* totally okay and should really be kept under wraps and in the dark.

For five years of our marriage my husband and I were celibate except for one occasion which took place in broad daylight, on a sheepskin rug in front of the fire and in the middle of a Saturday afternoon. What on earth would Reverend H and his wife have said about that! Yet God wonderfully blessed this union with the conception of our beautiful, perfect daughter, so *God* obviously sees nothing wrong with well lit, fireside sex on a Saturday afternoon!!

Hey! Did I just write that? "God *blessed* our union"? God blesses sex? Does He? I've got to think about that one! Satan uses it and spoils it but God blesses it. Isn't that the right way round? How then do I turn around the way I think and feel? Is it possible?

I remember early on in my psychotherapy telling Dr. Kapp about this long period of celibacy. I rattled on about the fact that my babies woke a lot during the night for feeds and nappy changes; they were a bit fidgety in bed, so it was easier for Frank and I to sleep in separate rooms. I slept in the double bed with baby daughter and Frank slept in the next bedroom with toddler son. That way we did manage to get a lot more rest.

I explained to Dr.Kapp that we never, in five whole years, found a spare moment for sex. We were busy parents and it was impossible. Our kids

THE HUDDLE

wouldn't let us. We didn't even share a bed. Et cetera. Et cetera. Dr. Kapp sat there listening as I went on and on and on. When I'd finally finished giving her this elaborate explanation which I though was quite convincing, she very calmly told me that she didn't buy a word of it! Ah well... For me, celibacy was fine, the answer to my difficulties and the perfect form of contraception. It meant that I could feel I was no longer performing for the devil, but it hardly suited Frank!

I don't want to write any more about occult stuff, but I hope I've written enough to indicate to you how it continues to put me off sex and make it extremely distressing for me. Apart from the memory thing and the flashbacks, I remain convinced that enjoying an active sex life belongs to the devil, and one of the things Satan does not want is for me to enjoy sex within the safe confines of marriage. That is, within God's rules and with His blessing. Wrong sex is right with Satan and right sex is wrong. He will do everything within my mind and spirit to spoil it and make it nigh on impossible for me.

It says in the Bible that God expects us to be in control of ourselves at all times, and as I see it, orgasms would belong to the out-of-control orgies of witchcraft. This is pleasure with the devil that pleases the devil and I believe I can only ever come close to God if I abstain from sex or at least gain no pleasure from it. God sees all. I can't bear Him seeing me doing that!

I have already dealt briefly with the Reverend H's attitude towards sex, but how about the rest of the church on earth? Churches that idolise, worship and venerate the Virgin Mary do not exactly help matters for twits like me. Mary, the Virgin Mary, is seen as pure, clean and unspoiled because she'd not had sex before Jesus was born. (I bet she did afterwards when she married Joseph!) So when God chose a woman who was good enough to have His son, then she had to be a virgin. Untouched by a man. Why? Are women who have a sex life somehow unclean and less acceptable to God? Does God prefer a virgin chaste and pure? Are celibate priests and nuns able to enjoy a closer union with God *because* of their lack of a sex life? Or are they secretly obsessed with the lack of it – rather like the anorexic is obsessed with thoughts of the food she will not eat?

I feel unclean due to sex. Dirtied by Satan, dirtied by rape, and spoiled. My husband is married to damaged, inferior goods. As Reverend H pointed out, my virginity should have been a precious and special gift to my husband on the night of our marriage. How quaint! – And thanks a lot, mate. How cruel and unfeeling of you to say this! I had no choice whatsoever when my virginity was torn out of me.

I wish I could build inside my heart an altar to God, and upon it burn all the memories of my encounter with the occult. Maybe then the words that the apostle Paul wrote to the Romans would come true for me. "And the God of peace shall bruise Satan under your feet shortly." (Romans 16:20) But Lord, don't just bruise the devil! Destroy him completely and eradicate him from every area of my life. May he no longer hound me, torment me or have any influence over me ever again.

THE HUDDLE

"...whatsoever things are pure, whatsoever things are lovely ... think on those things." (Philippians 4:8)

On to The Huddle now, then. The effects of The Huddle on my sex life are worse than all the other categories I have dealt with rolled into one! Why? Because they are in the here and now and are happening to me all the time. They are present in the present. Rape is, literally, in the past, as is the Reverend and occult dabbling. They are not, literally, happening to me now, day in, day out. The Huddle are with *me* constantly and are capable, willing and deliriously happy to be always reminding me of the miseries of the past. They imitate Reverend H and all his hurtful, damaging words. They show me the faces of rapists and imitate their voices and all the other noises that go with an act of rape. They pretend to be members of a coven that are watching me, watching, watching, watching, forever bloody watching……..

I do not intend to go into explicit details, I wish I had the courage to do so as to write it all out might help me, but I will try to give a brief outline of the misery The Huddle can cause in this area of my marriage.

It will begin well before bedtime when The Huddle will start tormenting me with the possibility that I will have to engage in 'that' when I go to bed.

"He gonna rape you again girlie! Who's gonna f**k the little darling tonight then? Who's gonna STINK with all that revolting SPUNK oozing out of you fat f………." Like that only also much worse. So much worse. Can't write it down.

Little wonder that I hate going to bed and will plan to go either before or after my husband in the hope of avoiding the sometimes inevitable. The Huddle will become more obscene and verbal as soon as we are in bed together and if we do have 'that' then they will verbally drool and dribble over every detail. And I mean *every* detail! EVERY LITTLE MINUTE, BLOODY DETAIL!!! It is obscene, humiliating, grotesque and no doubt potentially capable of driving one insane. One. Or two. Or three, or........

When 'that' is over, The Huddle will always, without fail, immediately begin calling me names. A dirty bitch. A slut and a whore. Satan's little f**k bag. Et cetera. Post coitus they will be at their loudest and most tormenting, reducing the event to an act of prostitutional sluttery with the devil himself. Animals rutting, out of control. I am being raped by anyone and everyone. People are watching me, even people I know. The Huddle are still watching like a bunch of leering, dirty old men, pimps, perverts, paedophiles, handling themselves as they watch and feeding on the action. Sex is for Satan. Food for the devil. They will be commenting, gawping, talking, shouting, enjoying, slobbering and jeering. Why should I have to do something that causes The Huddle so much pleasure? That surely can't be right. They are feeding off my sex life and gaining strength from it for God's sake! I would be wiser and better off never doing 'that'.

I rarely get more than one or two hours sleep during any night when 'that' has taken place. Usually I will come downstairs and either cry on the floor, pressing my hands over my ears, or else,

THE HUDDLE

better still, I will put my headphones on and listen to music in an effort to tune out of The Huddle. More often than not I end up taking some Largactil with a handful of painkillers…….

I don't want to write any more on this subject because I am getting too upset and angry and sorry for myself, which isn't helpful. So use your imagination if you must. You now know enough about The Huddle to have gained an inkling of what their obscene company and interference must be like. How would *you* cope with it? Would you still want to have sex with all that going on? Do you blame me for trying hard to avoid it?

Why can't my husband be an unselfish partner for once and make a decision with me to be celibate? Could he not do that to spare me just a little of all this suffering? Is it really too much to ask?

Sometimes I have very wrong and wicked thoughts. Like saying to my husband that I will only agree not to kill myself if he will give up using my body for his pleasure. That would be a sort of blackmail, I know, and then again, if I hate my life so much, then what does it matter what the hell anyone does to me?? My life does not seem to be worth the effort of making any part of it more acceptable and less distressing.

Do you know, I often feel guilty because I breathe! Air is valuable and I should not be taking up any of it. The Huddle are right. My life is a total waste and of no value whatsoever. The Huddle! Foul fiends of hell! Filthy obscene perverts!!

"The words of the Lord are pure words: as silver tried in a furnace of earth, purified seven times."

(Psalm 12:6) The words of The Huddle are not pure words. "The Lord shall cut off all flattering lips, and the tongue that speaketh proud things: who have said, with our tongue we will prevail." (Psalm 12:3&4) O Lord, why do The Huddle prevail? Why?? They say, "Our lips are our own: who is lord over us?" (Psalm 12:4) Angel replies that Jesus is Lord over The Huddle, and they do not reply to that.

I do not know what to make of that sentence – Jesus is Lord over The Huddle – what does that mean exactly? That He is in control of them? If that is so, and He loves me, then why does He not take them away from me or at least stop my ears from hearing them? I don't understand.

Sex, thank God, is not the only part of married life. There are plenty of other parts and unfortunately The Huddle will try and interfere in these also. However, I seem finally to have gained something of an upper hand in this and will no longer be goaded into rowing and arguing with Frank over the most trivial of things, on any occasion and under the slightest provocation. We very rarely have a row these days and although I can still hear what The Huddle are saying about Frank, and what they tell me to say and do to him, I am able to keep dumb about it, locking it away inside of me instead of exploding into an outburst that will upset all of us. That's what The Huddle want to happen.

The Huddle hate my husband. It is very difficult for me to live this way. They tell me every day that he hates me, he has never loved me, I hate him and I do not love him. Often I get very confused,

THE HUDDLE

almost believing The Huddle and becoming cold and indifferent towards the man I am married to. Frank does understand what is happening but this does not make it any easier for him to live with. It is an unacceptable situation and extremely awkward and sad. Not write any more now. Please, no more. I want to change the subject again.

Dr. Kapp came again this week and upon reading what I'd written about another psychiatrist in a previous chapter, expressed some degree of annoyance. She seems to think I have a 'thing' about her fellow professionals, especially other psychiatrists. I tend to be hostile towards them and maybe compare them with Dr. Kapp. Well, true and false!

Of course I felt hostile towards the other psychiatrists who have seen me! Take a look at it from my point of view! I did not know any of them. I did not want to see them. They were complete strangers who expected me to reveal our inner life to them. Their visits were forced upon me. Or else! Or else my husband would have me sectioned into St. Cadoc's. He threatened me with this for a very long time, claiming that as my husband he had the right and the power to do this dreadful thing. I did not realise at the time that he possessed no such right or power! So I was forced and threatened into seeing these other psychiatrists and, under these circumstances, what good did they do me? What good *could* they do me?? All three of them left me in floods of tears after their visits and more determined than ever to carry out a successful act of suicide. I found it all very negative and very abusive.

In case Dr. Kapp thinks otherwise, I never compared these psychiatrists professionally with the silly old bag. I couldn't!! I've known her for years, I knew the others for less than a few hours, if that. They were working for the NHS, doing a job. Dr. Kapp, I have always believed, was directed by God to spend time with me because she is a Christian, and that's totally different! At least it should be! God will have directed her into the type of work that she does and for me that *has* to be profoundly important. Why am I writing about this? Because it's something else I want to get off my chest, that's why. Good enough reason. My book anyway. I can write what I like. You still there, dear reader?.......

The thing is, up until this week I've found it very useful to have Dr. Kapp's comments on this crazy book, but after her 'rattiness' over a few things I have written (which she would no doubt deny – justifying her words with clever professional speak) I feel I have lost her much valued comments. I don't want her to read any more of my book, and that leaves me feeling oddly vulnerable. I can't cope with her getting 'ratty' again! I hate it! I hate the guarded look that comes over her face if I should dare to mention another member of her peculiar profession. Fiddlesticks and knickers…….

All day long, every day, I have them, The Huddle. *They* are always annoyed at me, stern with me and 'ratty' with me. And so much more and worse. Therefore I cannot bear *anyone*, least of all Dr. Kapp, to display even the minutest trace of, or

THE HUDDLE

comparison with, their sort of behaviour. I cringe when my kids squabble. I curl up inside when Frank raises his voice. I fall silent and want to cry when my shrink is not happy about something I have said or written. Feeling that most of the world is against me, anyone who claims they want to help me naturally comes under the utmost suspicion. Remember Reverend H? "A psychiatrist won't help you, Janet!" It has consequently taken years for me to arrive at the degree of trust I now have in Dr. Kapp. Now I'm bloomin' annoyed with her – but I'm not allowed to be…..

The Huddle are back in the desk lamp today and I have it turned on even though it is daylight. I'm hoping the heat of the bulb will burn them and cause them the greatest pain and discomfort. Light. The light of the world. Jesus. They hate that. Good!! They are telling me to stop typing now.

"You write the biggest load of f**king rubbish we….."

"Yes, wretched voices. I am well aware that this book is a load of rubbish. It's mostly about YOU and I so it would have to be RUBBISH wouldn't it!!"

It is boring, discursive, a waste of time and not worth the effort of keeping alive. It is like me. This book is me. I am the rubbish that it is.

"F**king right! Stupid bitch is…."

Janet Cooper

Lord, please, I do not want to go to bed tonight. If my husband wants to……. Lord, please???????????…………

THE HUDDLE

CHAPTER ELEVEN WHAT OF THE FUTURE??

When I came to write this last chapter I wanted it to be a glorious one, full of hope, courage, a willingness to face whatever life might throw at me, and encouragement to myself to go forward, whatever. But I am, at present, again very depressed and aware only of discouragement, of my many weaknesses and my lack of courage. Every glimpse of light merely makes the darkness I plunge back into even worse, and I realise that every time I claw my way back out of this darkness and once again feel light, warmth and hope, then I am closer to death. Better never to have seen the beautiful light than to remember it in a time of utter misery. Better by far to snuff out a life while there is light, rather than risk the return of such profound darkness.

The future is the ugly spectre I have reluctantly chosen to face by getting rid of my evil comforter and deciding to live. Lately I wonder if he's really left me, or am I deluding myself? Whatever the future may hold I know I should seek to allow it to happen, but I am not a courageous person and the bleakness ahead fills me with terror and an absolute dread that I dare not fully give thought to.

As I type these words I realise that I continue to be most painfully bereft at the loss of my comforter. Evil comforter, but evil for whom? I now have no comfort whatsoever should I dare give thought to the future. I must no longer cuddle us with the comfort of a way out, an ultimate pain relief if it all becomes even more unendurable.

I am no longer safe. I do not feel safe and wonder if my psychiatrist was right in imploring me to let go of the evil comforter. I am so confused about how I feel and how I *should* feel. "My soul chooseth strangling, and death rather than my life. I loathe it; I would not live always." (Job 7:15&16)

It is very difficult for us to think or write about the future while I identify so strongly with Job and cry out to God with him, saying, "Wherefore then hast thou brought me forth out of the womb? Oh that I had given up the ghost and no eye had seen me. I should have been as though I had not been. I should have been carried from the womb to the grave. Are not my days few? Cease then, and let me alone, that I may take comfort a little." (Job 10:18-20) In plain English, I wish I had never been born, I want to die, and I wish everyone would leave me alone to claim back my evil comforter and be comforted with the thoughts and knowledge of an end to my suffering.

If I look further than the end of any one day, then all I see is no end to the way that I am. More of the same. Hours, days, weeks, months, years of it. If I am honest to this book, and I might as well be, as the days of this year creep by, I am becoming more convinced that very soon I shall travel alone to Brecon and call back my evil comforter. Any evil comforter! There must be plenty of them, all ready and willing to latch on to somebody like us. I also know that I do not need to scramble back up to the Brecon Beacons to do this evil thing, although this is the one place I have

THE HUDDLE

heard silence. (I'll tell you about that in a minute or so) I know that it would indeed be a wrong thing to do, but I'm in hell anyway, so what's the point of carrying on like this? I am a burden to myself and a burden to my family. I have nothing to give any friend. I can contribute nothing useful to this pointless world. I do not view any life as precious and I bring no joy, no pleasure, no happiness and no benefit to any other human beings. My existence is of no value and does not glorify God in any way. This is no way to live!

Angel says "You MUST live, Janet!!" WHY??????? Then I read in Job chapter eleven. "Because thou shalt forget thy misery, and remember it as waters that pass away; and thine age shall be clearer than the noon day; thou shalt shine forth, thou shalt be as the morning. And thou shalt be secure, because there is hope; yea, thou shalt dig about thee, and thou shalt take thy rest in safety. Also thou shalt lie down and none shall make thee afraid; yea, many shall make suit unto thee. But the eyes of the wicked shall fail, and they shall not escape, and their hope shall be as the giving up of the ghost."

Lord, I do not believe all this! How can I when The Huddle deny it all the day long? Always I hear *their* voices. Seldom do I hear Yours. Me, and Jan, Rachel, Liz, Katy and little Janny – "They grope in the dark without light, and he maketh them to stagger like a drunken man." (Job 12:25) Staggering! Drunk with the words of The Huddle. There is no light for us.

Janet Cooper

Today is the 16th January 1997. It is only now, at 7.23p.m., that I am reasonably tuned out of The Huddle and left alone by the others. I have a thumping headache that has not responded to my many efforts to get rid of it, and I am also suffering excruciating period pain. I have been able to eat very little today due to feeling ill and because of the constant sickening comments The Huddle make. Liz burned yet another piece of toast under the grill. Rizzo the hamster died yesterday and The Huddle are accusing me of murder. Janny is upset and has been crying pitifully and unbearably.

"Where gone? A mousie gone? Where the mousie gone?"

She has played and cuddled the Rab Rab again and my left thumb is sore where she has been chewing and sucking on it.

I found myself in the bathroom this afternoon, smears of menstrual blood on my face and the taste of it in my mouth. I do not know which one of them is doing this. Rachel denies it emphatically. It is disgusting and revolting and I am so ashamed. The Huddle tell me to eat and drink my menstrual discharge. How absolutely sickening. I do not want to go on like this.

Rachel has been sat in my chair playing with the little present that Frank gave her for Christmas. She's lucky to be able to sit there; I can't at the moment because there are beetles in it and I am frightened and upset.

Not too long ago I found a note that Jan had written in work and stuffed in her uniform pocket. It went something like this-

THE HUDDLE

<u>VOICES</u>
Idiot!
Stupid bitch!
Creep!
Fat ugly cow!
We hate you!

This leads me to conclude that the elusive Jan also hears voices. Is there no one of us who is free of them? How does Jan cope with her voices? By the look of her, a lot better than I do! Then again, she's only around, as far as I know, for twenty or thirty hours a week to go to work. That's not so long to have to cope with it and I wish I only had The Huddle for that same number of hours each week!

Any minute now, the worms will emerge from the typewriter and I shall have to waste more time getting rid of them before I can carry on typing. It's all so time consuming! I could not pop to the post office today to post a parcel because I couldn't cope with dog muck on pavements.

"EAT IT!!" Today I can't face that command repeated over and over again until I can smell the stuff and taste it in my mouth and feel the texture on my tongue and the action of swallowing bloody dog s**t!

Today and for the next few days I am going to close my eyes every time I go to the loo and hope and pray I will not get blood on my hands or, worse, on my face.

"Lick it off! You filthy frigging bleeding ….. EAT IT!!!……" Et cetera.

The Huddle have been so close to me all day, passing their non stop commentary, gawping at me, smelling me and hating me.

"Stinking bleeding BITCH – she gonna bleed for days now, bleed and bleed and bleed and bleed and bleed and BITCH! BITCH!..."

I am thirty nine years of age and I could have many more years of this monthly increase in my misery. Perhaps because I am menstruating, I can feel myself today getting more and more depressed under the constant onslaught of the cruel Huddle. The thought of being alive a week from now fills me with infinite sorrow and it is right for Angel to keep reminding me to just get through today. Sometimes one more hour seems too much to bear.

Yet again I am dreading having to go to bed, having to lie there trying to get to sleep and hearing The Huddle from their place in the window. I am dreading my husband touching me and finding out that I am a bleeding pig. I am dreading being captive to the others' and feeling their various states of distress. I am dreading the long, dark hours, having to get up for some of them in a vain attempt to escape The Huddle. I am dreading being us for another night and dreading the dreams if they come, as they surely will. I am dreading waking up.

"Bitch is awake!"

I am dreading finding out that I am still alive in the morning and will have to face another day. What sort of a 'life' is all this?

I do not want my life. "God hath delivered me to the ungodly and turned me over into the hands of

THE HUDDLE

the wicked" (Job 16:11) and I cannot bear to live this way. But yet I have made a decision to live!!

I am chock-a-block full of conflicts and contradictions. I know that only in heaven will God wipe away all the tears from my eyes. There shall be no Huddle in heaven!

There is a city bright,
Closed are its gates to sin.
Nought that defileth,
Nought that defileth,
Can ever enter in.

Good! So no Huddle in heaven. I shall be forgiven and clean and lovely and I shall have no memory of my present state. To be with Christ, this is far better! I do not want to go on living as I do not see that I have a future.

So, close now to the end of this book, I realise that I shall not attain the hope expressed in the introduction. I had wanted, and still want, the last page to contain one glorious word. Silence! I do not have it, I want it, I long for it, and I would do anything to be free of The Huddle. DAMN THEM!!!!! I have experienced silence briefly and I want it back!

I think I've told you that I once experienced a period of silence. Perhaps now is a good time to explain how that came about. It was real, real silence as opposed to being tuned out of the voices but still aware of them and what they are saying.

What happened was this. I found myself in what I suppose must sound like an unusual situation. On a glorious summer's day last August I was up a mountain with a consultant psychiatrist sharing a tin of blackcurrant Tango and a bread roll. It didn't feel at all odd to either Dr. Kapp or myself, just very special and okay. I remember being overwhelmed with the fact that somebody thought I was worth taking out for the day and spending time with. How boring for Dr. Kapp and how wonderful for me! (And even more wonderful as I sit here, in my gloomy morbidity, is the fact that by beginning to recount this day, I already feel a shot of light into my depressed state! Thanks Elinor!)

I cannot remember exactly *how* this trip came about, but following something we'd been discussing, Dr. Kapp offered to take me to the Brecon Beacons for a day and I would leave my evil comforter there. I had not wanted to leave him close to home.

So off we went – me jokingly asking Dr. Kapp if there was enough room in her car for all of us! (I am able to display something of a sense of humour at times!) First of all we visited a little church in the middle of the quaint little town of Brecon where three of us (two plus Rachel) were entranced by the most beautiful stained glass window depicting Jesus with outstretched arms. There He was, looking at us, with us, and inviting us to Him. Stunning! Then following lunch we became gloriously lost in a maze of tiny roads before finally discovering a suitable mountain up which to climb.

We got as far up as we could and sat down. All of us. After catching my breath I got down to the serious business of reading out a prayer I had written down the night before; a prayer that

THE HUDDLE

committed my evil comforter to God, leaving him there on the mountainside for God to deal with in His way. I refused to keep him with me and he went.

Then we prayed and took communion together. Blackcurrant Tango and a bread roll, all perfectly acceptable to God whose Son assures us that where two or more are gathered together in His name, then He is there in the midst of them. (Matthew 18:20) Dr. Kapp and I were two *bodies*, but more than two people and it did not feel strange or wrong for each one of us to come together in this way, in communion with each other and with God. (Days later, Rachel gave Dr. Kapp a card thanking her for being willing to spend time with us in this way. We had all, bar Jan and Janny, signed this card and it had taken days for all the signatures to appear.)

It was as Dr. Kapp and I took communion that I fell silent but I was not fully aware of it until we were walking back down the mountainside. Several times I asked Dr. Kapp to stop just for a moment, and listen, 'it's so quiet! I can't hear anything – isn't that wonderful? It's lovely isn't it! Listen! Listen to nothing, it's silence, it's so quiet, it's beautiful isn't it?'

And it was. Absolutely beautiful and I could have stood there forever.

The strange thing about this silence was that during it I had no awareness or memory of The Huddle whatsoever. I did not know what had stopped in order for me to experience this silence and it was as if I had never heard The Huddle and they had never existed in my life. It was only when

The Huddle returned that I remembered them, realising what I'd been missing, and marvelling that it *was* possible to be free of them! Today I'd been free for a short, short while. I had known peace and joy. Silence. And hope.

The Huddle returned to me as we drove down the little road away from 'our' mountain. I recognized them instantly but I was determined that they should not spoil such a lovely day. I swallowed down the tears as they threatened to spill from my eyes.

"Are you alright?" Dr.Kapp asked.

"Yes. Thanks. I'm fine." And I most certainly *was* fine! I was disappointed that my Huddle free time had been short, but more than well satisfied that I had done what I had set out to do and it had been a real blessing to all of us. The brief Huddle free moments had been a bonus that dared me to hope.

So where had The Huddle *been* for those wonderful silent minutes? I have two theories about my temporary Huddle free state. The first theory being that I wanted so much to get rid of them that my mind made an almighty effort to block them out and managed to succeed for a short while. A mixture of wishing, hoping, praying, denying their existence, enormous mental effort and selective amnesia. Would it be possible to continue this sort of desperately wishful mental effort on any long term basis? The other theory is that God shut them up for me in order that I might be able to think clearly and pray away my evil comforter. I believe with all my heart that Jesus was present in a very real way up there on that mountain and The Huddle

THE HUDDLE

could not dare to be too close to Him. They hate Him and are terrified of Him, so it would make sense for them to scurry away when He was so close to Dr. Kapp and the rest of us.

Moments after Dr. Kapp had prayed and we took communion I started to 'hear' this silence, as if Jesus had stilled all noise, everything, driving all evil away with His presence so that we could all come to Him unhindered and in a precious and special way. A communion of souls that was out of this world. The Tango and the bread were the wonderful symbols that God accepted, honoured and blessed, and how blessed we were on that day. Our communion with Him went far deeper than I am capable of expressing and I'm sure will influence far more people than just the group of us who gathered on that mountain. It was a rare experience.

When I came home that day I was elated and filled with love. I knew that I had done the right thing and my feelings towards my family changed dramatically for the better and I *knew* that I loved my children so very much. Knowing that I had made the decision to live somehow freed me to express this love and feel it as a new and living emotion. I felt so much relief, although at times I was to become bereft at the loss of my comforter.

This 'bereftness' plus my periods of depression seem to suggest I have turned my back on that glorious day, following which I looked forward to more times of 'silence' which did not happen. There have been no more experiences of those wonderful Huddle free moments and I still have the damn voices ALL the time. Tormented without further reprieve!

I AM HEARING VOICES ALL THE TIME, EVERY DAY, AND I THINK THAT I SHALL GO MAD!!!!!!!!!!!!!!!!!!

That day has not lost its power! Amazingly, telling you about this day is to re-live its profound effect upon us all. The sun shone, we were valued and cared for, Jesus was so very real and close, and I remember vividly the way I had felt during my time out with Dr. Kapp. This book may not end with the word I had wanted it to end with, but at least now it will not end with the hopeless gloom that has invaded this last chapter.

I can this very minute see an alternative to my repetitive need to plan my death. That is, to *accept* the way that I am. I would be better off to accept that I have The Huddle, I might always have them, and so I might as well make the best of it. This does not mean I shall give up wishing I didn't have them, or give up the struggles of each day. They will no doubt continue to make me depressed from time to time. But to end my life would mean that they had won. They never will!

The mountain and the Tango and the bread roll are a profoundly helpful memory of a past event. Jesus is not a memory; He is just as real and remains ever present. He is just as available to me now as He was on that day, and His light will still shine just as brightly, however dark my mind.

And about Dr. Kapp – I did not hear her silent prayers that day. But I believe deep within my heart

THE HUDDLE

that she placed each one of us into the care of God, not for that day only, but forever. Now, as I type, I am saturated in her prayers for me and for all of us. A light has once again been turned on, bringing the hope that yet another depression is on its way out. Another light at the end of another tunnel. That's why I shall live. Maybe one day I shall thank Dr. Kapp, Elinor, for saving my life… Till then,

I SHALL NOT GIVE UP, EVEN WHEN DISMAYED, FOR I *HAVE* FOUND GOD!!!

Lord I believe, help thou mine unbelief.
AMEN.

Janet Cooper

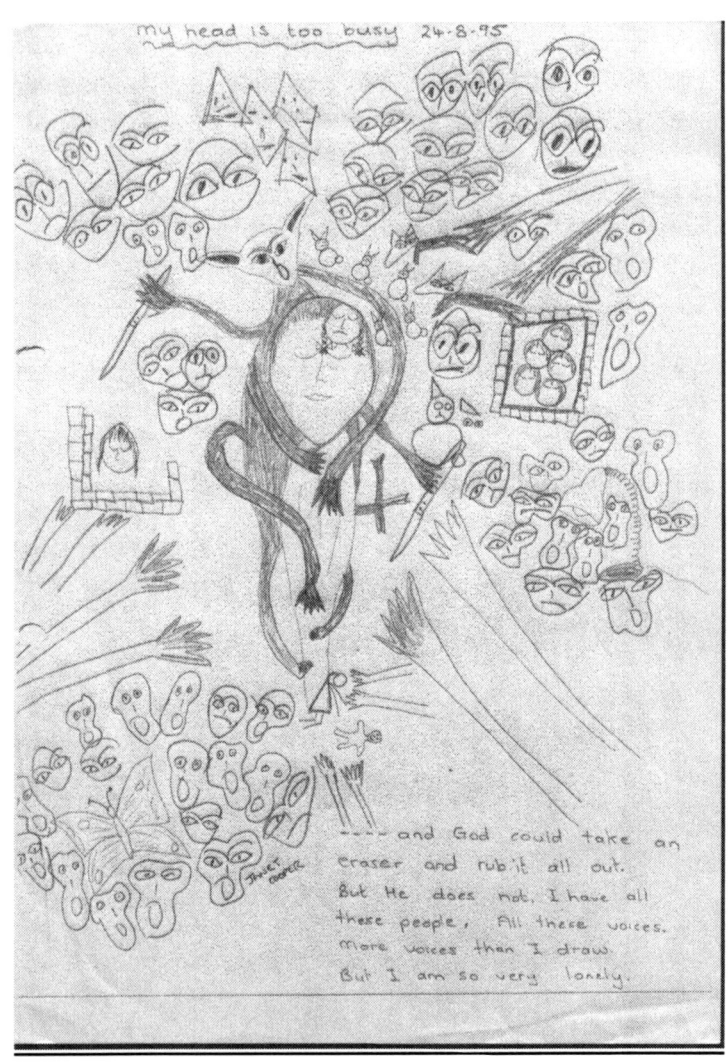

THE HUDDLE

ABOUT ME AND MY VOICES

Rachel

Janet Cooper

THE HUDDLE

INTRODUCTION

My name is Rachel and Janet said I could write a book about my voices when she had finished the one about The Huddle so now she has finished it is my turn.

We have been trying to work out how we would do it. I wanted to type it myself but I don't really like typing and can't do it fast like she can. Then we thought that I could be telling her what to type while she is typing it but we have now worked out that the best way is for me to write down what I want to say and she will type it out for me and then all the capital letters and things like full stops will be in the right places. She has promised not to change what I say but I don't mind it if I spell something wrong and she puts it down right. She has said will I not go on about sex and being raped and that sort of thing, but if this is my book, I want to write what I like. She said it would all get typed! She also said I better not write anything about other doctors because if I show my book to Elinor she will get her hair off again. Sometimes I think Elinor is pretending to be a school teacher.

If Janet does not type down everything that I want to say then I think I will get very angry and will have to type it myself in secret. And I *can* do that. So there!

I want to write lots of chapters like Janet did. I have never tried to write a book before. I do not think it will be a very long one but she says that does not matter. I don't know if I can do this but Angel says to try.

Janet Cooper

Janet says I have got to write as if I have a pretend reader. She says to pretend I am telling it all to someone and write just like I would talk.

We had a row about one thing and that is that I wanted my book in a file all by itself but Janet wants to put it in with her book so that it will be all like one book about us. I would have liked *my* book to be first but it does not matter. I am very excited about doing this so I do not really care. I don't care now. I have got a very bad headache again today and I am going to call my first chapter 'WHO AM I?'

Here goes then. I hope that you like reading my book.

THE HUDDLE

CHAPTER ONE   WHO AM I?

Hello. My name is Rachel. I do not have a surname or a middle name. I have always been only Rachel. I live behind the face of someone but I am somebody else. I am me and I have always been me.

I think I am a bit of a funny 'me' because now I am all jittery and flittery, like a very worried little sparrow that does not know what is going to happen to it. If I tweeted like a bird, it would be a very sad little tweet and I do not feel very good about myself but I am always me.

Some people have thought that I am other things and not me. Frankie (Janet's husband) said I was a voice and for a long time he thought I was evil and I should go away. The worst of all was the Rev who said I was a demon and kept telling me to go to hell and the pit and Gehenna. He really did my head in! He called me names like demon, evil spirit, wicked creature, evil thing, and one of Satan's little minions. He said I was pathetic and that he hated me, god hated me, and the whole of heaven hated me. I went nuts!

Elinor has said words to describe me like I am an auditory hallucination. I know what that means. It means hearing a voice that isn't really there, but I *am* really here! I am *not* a voice in Janet's head, I am *me*! Silly old bag, but I like her lots. Then she rattled on about an alter ego and another persona. I know what all that means as well. I am *not* an alter ego or another persona; I am a separate 'I'.

Then Elinor said I was a split off bit of Janet's personality. That was a bit of a cheek to say that and I did not like being described as a split off 'bit'! Even sillier old bag!! I am *not* a bloody split off '*bit*', I am ME!

Then one day Dr. Sami came because Janet had swallowed too many tablets and I told him to get lost when he tried to put a thing around her arm to take her blood pressure and then I told him to f**k off (oops! But I don't care!) and threw a pillow at him. He then said I was another personality, which is really quite right because that means that I am another person. I AM ME! I am Rachel. I think they all realise that now.

I am seventeen years old. I always have been and I don't have any birthdays, I do not know why, that is just the way it is for me because when Janet was younger than seventeen she needed someone older to look after her and tell her what to do. I used to be very bossy indeed. Then when she got to be older than me, it was not so good and I got quite nasty for a long time. I was my nastiest when we were seeing the Rev.

I think I have always been here but I can't remember very much about Janet being younger than eight, I think I can remember only that far back.

I am a girl. It is not always very easy to share a body. We get ill at the same time with colds and things like that, and we have our periods together but sometimes I am depressed when Janet is not and that can work the other way round as well, but when one of us is depressed for a few days, the other one catches it and we both end up the same.

I was very frightened when Janet was having her babies and I did not want anything to do with it

THE HUDDLE

all. I hid away and I was scared. She let them suck on her tits and I did not want to know because I did not like the babies. But I do now. I think the two chickadees are brilliant and I like them lots and lots. I talk to them but they don't know it is me and Janet does not seem to know it is me either, and today Janet was going to Tesco's with Heather for shopping and Heather said she had to go to the loo and I said 'Me too!" and we had a race up the stairs and we were both laughing. I got there first and had a wee first and Heather thought it was really funny. They like it when I squeal loud and talk a bit silly but I don't always feel like doing that. I have got used to them calling me 'Mum' and I don't really mind.

It is very funny, but Janet did not know what my name was until about seven years ago and I never told her because she never asked me. She just knew that I was here and I would talk to her and she would talk back, all inside our head, and she never bothered about calling me a name.

My name has always been Rachel and when the Rev thought I was a demon and tried to get rid of me, he said, "What is your name? Give me your name!" Straight away I said "Rachel" because that is my name. I am Rachel. "No", he said, "Give me the name by which you are known in hell!" I kept telling him I was Rachel but he did not believe me and I got very upset and ill and I had a big one of them nervous breakdown things and we went to hospital twice. We hated it. I hear voices as well but I don't call mine The Huddle.

I live in the very, very middle of this head in a bare room that we call my cell. When Janet was very depressed and I was driving her mad and she wanted to get rid of me, she used to build lots and lots more bricks round and round me to block me in and shut me up and try to make out I was not here. I got angry and screamed a lot and cut her. I was scared, then Elinor persuaded Janet to let me have a window, and one day she did, so I can look out when I like, but mostly I curl up on the floor in a corner or lie down, all curled up. Elinor said to decorate my grey breeze block cell to make it pretty for me but I can't do that because I think it should be bare and miserable. I think I am punishing myself for being a witch and I did some bad things. Being alive feels very horrible now. I did put a curtain over my window and I close it when I want to be alone and private. Then Janet knows she shouldn't talk to me. Sometimes when I am in a very bad mood I swish it shut and I sulk. It is a yellow curtain with pretty flowers on it.

I hope you know who I am now. Just because I share a body, it does not mean that I am not a real person. I am me. ME! ME!! ME!!! I AM RACHEL. I have a name. I can talk and do things. I can think. I *do* have feelings. I cry a lot these days and I never used to. I thought it was childish to cry and I was too strong to do it. Sometimes when I cry when Elinor is here, she gives me a hug and I cry some more and then I feel a bit better. She says that she likes me. Nobody has ever told me that before.

Who am I?   <u>I AM RACHEL!!!</u>

THE HUDDLE

CHAPTER TWO   A BIT ABOUT ME AND JANET AND... THE OTHERS

Janet hates me. She says that she doesn't hate me any more and tries to be nice to me, but I don't believe her and I don't trust her. She doesn't trust me either. Ages ago she wrote an essay which shows how much she hates me and wishes I was not here. She would like to get rid of me but knows that she can't. I got the essay out of her diary and she said she would type it out for me when I asked her. This is it.

A RACHEL FANTASY

Rachel couldn't understand how they had broken into her cell. It had seemed so secure. So complete. So utterly captive making. So endless. So terrible. So lonely. Oh! So very, very lonely! But, after all, how her imprisonment was justified! She was evil and had done awful things. She deserved to be out of the way, but how she longed for someone to talk to. Tell them how she felt. Be held safe.

And now here were two people, a man and a woman, breaking into her cell. She didn't know them and they knew very little about her. The man had never even met her! This wasn't how she had wanted her captivity to end. Not in this violent way with herself totally out of any control of the situation. She supposed they thought her to be psychotic. She supposed dead right! Intractably depressed. Malignantly suicidal. Rachel knew that all three descriptions described her pretty accurately. Her miserable enforced state. She began to whimper and to moan.

As they came into her cell through the smashed rubble, Rachel crouched into a grey, breeze block corner. They inched slowly towards her as if she was a dangerous animal about to spring. Dr. Huge, the man, slightly depressed the plunger of the glass syringe he held before him like a threat. It yielded a shower of little demons which held Rachel mesmerised with fear as Dr. Black caught hold of her arm, none too gently. Before she could do anything, Rachel felt the needle pierce the skin of her upper arm and she let out a primitive howl. Dr. Huge and Dr. Black had captured her. Captured her in her captivity. And shall captors lead captives free? Not this side of heaven!

Rachel was bundled into the back of a large grey car and taken to St. Lucifer's. She was lead, drowsy now and hardly able to walk, down a long, long corridor at the end of which was a treatment room. Treatment for Rachel. She passed an office whose door stood wide open and inside sat Mrs. Shrink. There were toys on the floor and Rachel tried to go in. She wanted to play. Wanted to talk. But no. too old now to play with toys.

"Go away, Rachel. I'm busy with Janny!" Said Mrs. Shrink.

Rachel was told to lie on a bed in the treatment room and she felt too lethargic and despairing to put up much of a struggle as they fastened leather straps around her wrists, ankles and body. She could hear Dr. Huge talking to Dr. Black.

"Yes! ETC. I think it might be worth a try ... no, she won't need an anaesthetic, Rachel doesn't feel

THE HUDDLE

pain. Look at her arms, cuts, didn't feel them. Not possible to hurt Rachel."

Rachel lay there. Speechless. Past caring. This really was the end. She could feel herself finally giving up and giving in to them. The end. No more. PING! Oblivion. She began to utter a prayer to her master.

"I pray to thee O Satan...."

Dr. Huge and Dr. Black placed the electrodes on her scalp.

"...to make it painless, make it quick..."

They checked the voltage on their equipment.

"...take me, kill me, help me..."

Dr. Huge threw a switch. The current surged and hummed.

"Please just end it for me. End, end, end, end..."

Rachel's body convulsed violently. Too violently. As Satan himself leapt through the wires, entering her damaged soul and possessing her for ever and ever and ever and ever and ever......

The end had only just begun.

Janet sat at home while all this was going on, and ate another prune covered in natural yogurt. Low fat, of course. It coated the plump, juicy fruit like a pure white emulsion. White covering black. Good against evil. Light chasing out the darkness. RUBBISH! Yogurt covering a prune, that's all!

Janet ate it slowly, very slowly. Then, as delicately as possible, she plopped the stone out of her mouth and onto the little teaspoon. Carefully, deliberately, daintily, she placed the sucked stone onto the pretty bone china plate beside her. She looked at it. Couldn't help staring at it. Seemed daft, but that's how it was. The stone sat there. It was hard and unyielding. Defiant. It was also useless to Janet. It needed to be got rid of. She didn't want it. Throw it away. Put it in the bin. Out with the rubbish. Out! OUT!! It had sort of sharp edges to it. Cutting edges. Pain causing edges. Honed and hard. A stone. It was only a stone damn it! But it reminded Janet of.....

Janet felt annoyed that she didn't seem able to taker her eyes off it.

Suddenly!
Loudly!!
Mockingly!!!..........

"Hello!" Said the stone. "I'm Rachel! Swallow me......"

THE END OF RACHEL'S FANTASY
I think that this story proves that she hates me and does not want me here.

("Rachel! That was written a few years ago!"
"Well?"
"Things are different now and at least I've been trying to get on with you a bit better!"
"I know, but you still don't want me, you still wish I wasn't here, I know you do, I'm not stupid!")

Janet still does not want me and would like not to have to share with me. We talk quite a lot inside our head and I suppose that most of it is okay and not really bad but we both tend to remember the bad bits most of all, like when we have hurt and

THE HUDDLE

upset each other. Janet is now much better at letting me share doing things when I want to. Elinor told her to. I like to read some of the things she reads and I like listening to music with her. It drowns out the voices. Bach and Mozart are alright but we like Status Quo and Boney M and Elton John, which isn't too bad, but Heather is really into the Spice Girls and I like them a lot. But a lot of the time I feel too miserable to want to do anything and I pull across my curtain and curl up with my arms around my head. Often all I want to do is watch and look and listen to what is going on.

Me and Janet argue a lot about things such as do we have a shower or a bath, who will make the beds (I make them neater than she does) and about what we are allowed to wear and eat. Sometimes I make the effort to come out and be here on my own and then I can do what I like but I don't stay only me for long because it makes me very tired and scared. I am frightened of being in the world and living. It is not good. It is bad.

I know about the others that are here as well as me. I think there are two more than what Janet has written about. I do not know if she knows about them or not. I don't care, but I think that Jan would know because she knows everything.

I think Liz is the one I hate the most because she is so nasty. Lots of times she cut our breasts and then there was a lump that came and I stuck a knife in it and yellow stuff came out. It is better now but there is still a lump but Janet says it does not matter so we don't care about it. The scars are very sore and hurting. It was Liz's fault.

Janet Cooper

Liz has a room with a big bed in it. There is a dressing table in front of a window and a built in wardrobe in an alcove by the side of a fireplace. She is sixteen and a pain in the backside. I have tried to make friends with her but she does not want to know me. She sits with her eyes tight shut and keeps banging her leg with her hand and calling everyone nasty and saying she doesn't care about anything. She says she is going to swallow lots and lots of slug pellets. She is like a spaggy cat and I wish she was not here.

Katy also has a bedroom and since Elinor came she has a nice bed in it and a rug on the floor and pretty curtains. She spends most of her time lying on the bed either totally silent or else cry and screaming her head off. The screaming drives me nuts and makes *me* feel like screaming as well!

Janny drives me round the bloody twist. She's like a whiney little kid who won't shut up. I don't know if she has a bedroom. She sucks her thumb and her hand. She makes stupid little noises and keeps calling things by baby names, like 'rab rab' for rabbit, and 'mouses' for the gerbils and hamster. Only one hamster now because Rizzo died. I liked him. He was cute. I don't like Janny, she gives me the creeps, I do not think that she is normal.

If I want to I am able to talk to Liz and Katy but not to Janny, she does not seem to hear me or take any notice. Katy takes notice of me because I am older and I have been teaching her some hymns on the piano. Can't teach her much else because Janet ripped the music books up. Hate her for that. Sometimes I play the piano and Katy sings. We like

THE HUDDLE

doing that and nobody knows it's us and not Janet, so we can do it when we want to.

I have Angel as well and I think she talks to me more than she talks to Janet. I also sometimes have Jesus in my head but nobody believes that. He is a light, and I want to go towards the light because then I would be better.

I don't know Jan but I know that she is here. She is over all of us. She goes to work. I am not allowed to have anything to do with Jan going to work and Janet being with her because the Rev said I was dangerous, like full of evil and so Janet wants me out of the way in case I try to be here on my own for a few hours when they are in work. This used to get me very upset but now I don't mind so much because I don't want to be anywhere else anyway!

One night when they were in work I tried to fight my way out. I wanted to see what was going on and to watch and listen. Janet realised what I wanted to do and tried to stop me. Then it all went wrong, all upset and exploding inside us and then Janet was on the floor and throwing up and had a severe throbbing headache. She could not move her head or open her eyes because the pain was so bad. A doctor sent her to hospital in an ambulance and we were there for two days and they said that she had a severe migraine attack. Janet said it was my fault, that I was stressing her out. I don't think that is fair.

Nearly every day we have a headache, and at one time Liz was having terrible headaches, all sickey, and we felt them as well and were ill with them. It was horrible.

Although there are a few of us here, I feel very, very lonely. It would be nice to have a really, really friend but I don't think I am nice enough. I used to swear an awful lot. Bad words. But in the last few years I have stopped doing that almost completely. My swearing and my nastiness got worse when we were seeing the Rev. He kept telling me I was evil and I was a demon and so in the end I started acting like one. I was like he expected me to be. It took Elinor a long time to convince me I was not a demon because I had come to believe that I must be. Now that I know that I'm not, I do not have to act or swear like one.

When Janet was very depressed a few months ago and went to bed in the middle of the afternoon because she wanted to be dead, I made her get up and plant crocus bulbs. They are growing now and I am going to give every flower a nice name. Hope, joy, peace, love, gentleness............like that. Then they will be Jesus flowers and remind us of Him. They will be lovely colours like He is. Sometimes I see Him, see light, and I do not know what to do about it. I *know* Jesus. Not like I know Janet or Frankie or Elinor. I *know* Him. Like we are close and very together. He is the light that I see and when I am in the light, then He is in me. I can't say what I mean because I am not clever at describing it. I just know that I know Him.

I do not think that Jesus wants me to be a normal part of this world. But I am not abnormal or a witch or a demon either. I am me. I am Rachel. Rachel loves Jesus. Jesus loves Rachel. If He didn't then I would not be here. It is really very simple.

But lots of times I am in darkness and it feels very horrible and scary and we can hear Jesus on

THE HUDDLE

the cross and how much it hurt Him and we lie down and cry about it and feel as if we are dead too and we are going mouldy and rotten. It is very awful indeed.

I have been looking through her diary and she wrote this about me too.

<u>RACHEL</u>

Spiteful, spaggy, mocking, critical.
Her nag, nag, nag is intermittent,
Yet constantly so.
Through day, through night,
Too constant, but erratic,
Sporadic and sudden.
Expected always.
Threatening.,
Sometimes feared,
Sometimes oddly comforting.
Waited for,
Never far away.
Peace, perfect peace?
In heaven.
Only in heaven.
Then, and only ever then,
AMEN.

See? She doesn't like me, does she! I don't think Frankie does either, he just puts up with me because I am here. He treats me like a kid but I know Elinor likes me. I am going to copy Janet and write a chapter about our psychiatrist. I don't know if I'm doing alright with this book but it feels nice to scribble and scribble away about me.

I hear voices as well. One of them is the Rev and he keeps on and on and on when I am writing this. He is saying things like,
"Do you think God really wants you to write that?"
"Is this writing glorifying to God? I think not!"
"REPENT! And beg for forgiveness!"

The night before Janet went to St. Cadoc's for the first time he slapped her hand and called me a wretched sinner because I couldn't stop biting her hand. They were telling me to hurt her, the voices were. So I was trying to. I was very frightened and couldn't work out what was going on. Next morning, Mrs. Rev made us have a bath and she sat on the loo and watched us. That was horrible. Then she made us get dressed and a doctor came and we went straight to hospital. It was very cold and nasty there and I was very scared. They wanted to get rid of me. Scared and frightened and very cold.

I think this is the end of this chapter now because I am getting very tired.

"Are you sure?" (Janet)

Yes. I want to have an end by here now for today. I am very, very lonely. I wish I was in heaven. I am scared. I am Rachel.

THE HUDDLE

CHAPTER THREE   MY VOICES

My voices are very bad and they are in my cell with me all over the place and sound a lot as if they are inside my head. I do not call them a huddle because I think it is stupid to give them a name. I hear them through my ears, in the middle of my brain. I do not like them and I wish that I did not have them. I think that one day they will kill me. I put my hands over my ears a lot in the hope of blocking them out of my ears but it does not work.

They say bad things about me and they want to f**k me all…

"I am *not* typing this word for word!" (Janet)
"Why not? What's wrong now? You had all the bad words in *your* book!"
"I know, but…"
"BUT WHAT! I hate you; I really, really hate you! I hate you, I hate you, I hate you…"

(Janet speaking here! I have spoiled her book! I have, by the side of my typewriter, several sheets of Rachel's writing. They have been torn angrily to shreds. By me, and I'm sorry. I lost my temper. I have promised her I will type exactly what she puts in future, but now I have a major sulk on my hands. I do everything wrong!)

Me Rachel. Slow typer. Very upset. Don't want to talk. Me go away a bit now. Don't care. Janet's mother says that I am a nasty little cat. She is a voice in my head sometimes. There are other ones as well. Do not want to talk. Go away now.)

Janet Cooper

This is a few days later now. We had a very bad row and then yesterday Janet spent ages with me because I wanted to swallow lots of tablets. So did she. But she said maybe we should wait a bit before doing it so that I can finish my book. So I will write more today. About my voices. She says that she does not want me to write the dirty and nastiest bits in case one of the chickadees somehow gets hold of this and reads it. She said they would not understand and would be upset, but they know about me, that I am here, but I have said okay, I will not put certain things and words in my book. I don't really care. Doesn't really matter. Got to write about my voices again now.

I can give a better description about my voices than Janet gave about The Huddle. I think there are about twelve of them in a group and some are male and some are female and they've all got very hard, snarling sorts of voices as if they hate me, which they do.

Yes. There would have to be twelve because then with me as well that would make thirteen and that is a coven. That is what Satan would want. But I don't want to be part of them any more. I am not a witch now. The female voices also sound very hard and deep, like a man's, but I know that they are female.

I recognise one of the voices and that one is an exact copy of the Rev's voice. This is the worst voice of all because it is very loud and it keeps on at me all the time. It says things like the Rev said in real life, like about me being a demon, and hated, and it tells me to go all the time. Every time we walk through a door this voices says, like,

THE HUDDLE

"Go!"
"Get out!"
"Out in the name of Jesus!"

I think the Rev will be in trouble with God for the things he said to me and telling me to go to hell when Jesus loves me and wants me. That is very serious.

I feel that I have the Rev in my head all the time and that he is still trying to exorcise Janet and I am one of the demons he is trying to get rid of and I remember a lot of the screaming me and Janet did when he was holding her down and shouting at me to get out of her. I hate this voice most of all and I would like to kill myself to get away from it. It even looks like the Rev.

The voices are able to copy people I know and still know. They copy nasty people who did bad things and they copy Frankie and Janet's mother and Elinor, but it is always a very bad copy and they want to make me hate the people they are copying. Then if I do, they change back and tell me how bad and evil I am to hate people. I can't help it when they keep on all the time. Then they laugh at me a lot and they try to drive me mad. But I am not mad. I am me. I am Rachel.

All these voices are in my cell with me. If I am in one corner, they will be in another corner but I hear them in my head. I cannot escape from them and I get very frightened indeed. Very, very sometimes, when I have been out, they have come from the same places as The Huddle come from, but not very often as they are nearly always heard in my head even though I know they are on the other side of my cell. It is not very easy to describe but I know what I mean.

They say bad things to me. They are always telling me that I am stupid and ugly and they use a lot of very bad swear words like s**t and f**k and c**t and b*****d and a lot more. They say that I am an evil secret in Janet's head and nobody wants me. They say that nobody loves me, but Elinor loves me, she says she does and nobody has ever told me that on the whole of my life so then they say bad things and that she is a liar.

They laugh at me a lot, especially when I am very sad and crying. They laugh when I play the piano but it doesn't stop me playing like it used to. They are only jealous because they cannot play or sing nice tunes. I think they might be jealous because I am me and they are not.

I am trying not to swear or be bad any more, but *they* can't help swearing and being bad all the time. It must be horrible to be so horrible and not be able to stop. Jesus has not given them an angel in their heads like I have got.

I do not have lots of coping methods like Janet because my cell is bare but I do things with her that take my mind off the voices for a bit. I listen to music, try and read with her, I play the piano and help do things like mixing a choccy cake for the chickadees. I like it when she turns the tele on just so that I can sit on the settee and turn if off! It's great! I look at the screen and see people talking. Voices talking. Then I point the remote control at the voices and – ZAP!! – I turn them off! I love doing that. I pretend that I have a remote control in my cell and I aim it at the voices and try to turn

THE HUDDLE

them off but it only works with the tele. It is nice to pretend it works with the voices as well. It makes them laugh at me, but they laugh at me anyway so it does not really matter.

Sometimes I talk to Katy when she is upset. I don't like doing this, but if I don't she starts screaming again and that drives me nuts.

I hear Janet as a voice inside my head. Like the others. People, but voices inside my head because I cannot always see them when I talk to them. But I know what they look like and I do sort of see them but not like really seeing something outside yourself. Me and Janet can talk to each other a lot without using our throats or mouths because we only have one throat and one mouth between us, so we don't bother with them. It is not necessary for us to use a body in order to talk to each other. It is very easy, but we don't always want to listen to each other but often we can't help it.

I hear Angel. She is an angel but I hear her voice very deep in the middle of my head. She is the only voice that I have that only ever says nice and good things to me. When I am especially sad and lonely she sings this to me – I will write it down, it has a nice tune and I am going to learn it on the piano. This is it –

I heard the voice of Jesus say
Come unto me and rest.
Lay down, thou weary soul lay down
They head upon my breast.
I came to Jesus as I was,
Weary and worn and sad,
And found in Him a resting place,

Janet Cooper

And He has made me glad.

I do not *feel* very glad and as if I have a resting place, I am not glad but I like this hymn because it makes me think of Jesus as a nice voice when the others are so nasty.

Angel says things to me like Elinor says. Angel tells me that I am not a demon, nobody will get rid of me and send me to hell, and Jesus loves me. I do not always believe her but it is nice to hear all this. Her voice is very soft and gentle and serious and when she says something I can always hear her even above all the other voices. I think she is above them because she is an angel and they are not. I do not want to think about what they are. I do not want to know. They are just bad voices.

I have always heard voices. I cannot remember a time when we never did. They got very very much worse after we met the Rev. Often Janet used to pretend that she wasn't hearing voices any more just so that he would stop trying to exorcise her all the time, but he would know that she was lying because he could tell she was still hearing them. She turns her head to where they are and looks like she is listening to something and I think that used to show him that the voices were still there. Anyway, she could never pretend for more than a few days at a time because pretending made them worse and she did not know how to be someone who does not hear voices. She would try to be very happy that they had gone but it did not work because they had not gone and she was not happy in any way and she would end up worse than ever.

THE HUDDLE

I have never pretended that my bad voices have gone because they haven't and I think the only way to get rid of them out of my head is to kill myself but Elinor said to Janet on Monday that how would she know that she would not hear voices when she is dead. So maybe I would as well, and I think that is cruel because we all have to die one day and it is too bad to think we will never not hear them.

Me and Janet both believe that we will not hear bad voices when we are dead and it is very nasty for someone to say that we might. There are not any tears in heaven so there can not be any bad voices either because bad voices make you cry.

I will kill myself on a Wednesday because Dr. Sami does not work on Wednesday afternoons and he won't be able to send us to hospital to have our stomach pumped out and Frankie can't drive. Elinor says that if I kill myself then I will kill all of us but I don't see how she can be right. I don't think the others would mind anyway. It would be better than being how we are. I know that.

Sometimes I have done bad things that the voices have told me to do. I cut us with a knife and I stick pins in and squeeze blood out. Once I was making myself sick a lot and I hated that but they kept telling me to do it. When Janet took too many tablets one day when the chickadees went back to school I made us sick and saved her life. I don't know why, I think I was frightened that I would go to hell and the voices would come with us. All these mushy tablets came up, all white slimey stuff and it made my throat bad and my muscles in my tummy got very sore for days after. After I was sick she kept trying to take more tablets but the only ones left were not strong enough to kill her.

Other bad things that they have got me to do years ago was to go out on my own in the night and do bad things, and I did very bad things in the Rev's church and bad things for the devil that Satan kept telling me were really good things. Now I know that they weren't. Janet does not want me to put it all in her book but she says if I want to write about it then I can write to Elinor. So I will just say that I did a lot of bad things that the voices told me to do. I thought that terrible things would happen if I did not do as I was told. They said I had to be a good girl.

Hearing voices makes me cry a lot. I think it would be very nice not to be as we are and I would like to get rid of all the bad voices. I think that Elinor should be able to get rid of them because she is a psychiatrist, but she can't. I wish that she could. I have tried to wrap them all up in a brown paper parcel and give it to her to chuck away. I do this in my head. It does not work and they laugh at me.

I would not like to get rid of angel because she is very nice. It is horrible to have voices that say nasty things to you all day long and calling you bad names. They hate me, and now I hate myself. I did not hate myself before I met the Rev as I knew that Janet would not manage without me, but then he kept saying that she would, I was bad for her and I had to go. He is very bad for me and I hate him lots and even more now that he is a bad voice. I would like very much to write him a long letter telling him how wrong and bad he was and exactly what I think of him, but he would only think it was a letter from a demon and he would then say that

THE HUDDLE

Janet was still possessed and so I will not write such a letter. Pity really. I would love to get my own back on him for hurting me.

Sometimes I try to imagine what it would be like if I did not have these bad voices all the time. But I can't imagine it and I feel very jealous of people who can not hear them. I think they must be better people than we are. Elinor does not hear voices and sometimes I get angry about that and I want to hit her and tell her to get lost because she does not understand, but then I think maybe she does just a bit.

I would like to give the voices to people I do not like so that they have them and I don't. I think that most of all the Rev should have them so that he would know that people who hear voices are not mad or possessed by demons. Maybe then he would think that people who hear voices were special people, although it does not feel very special, it feels very bad and sad and mad. And it is very, very lonely, but we are never alone.

The voices are uninvited guests. What a bloody cheek! I damn well f**king hate the dirty f**king b*****ds and I'd like to kill them and stamp their bloody brains out and I hate them and hate them and I f**king s**tting arsehole hate them, swining bloody s**ts of b*****ds! I don't care and I bet you won't type that bit!!

Janet Cooper

(See Rachel? I have typed it. I *do* understand your anger and you wanting to express it this way.)

I did not invite the voices and I do not want them. I wish they would go away. I wish I did not hear voices. I talk to Jesus inside my head and ask

THE HUDDLE

Him to take them away but He doesn't. He still loves me though. When I wrote the bad words a few sentences ago the Rev said,
"Ah! See? A demon! Put away all filthy communication from out of your mouth! Do you think God wanted you to write that down?"
YES! I think that God *did* want me to write it down because He wants me to feel better and sometimes I feel better after writing all the bad down. Why doesn't God make me better?
My voices are very bad.

("Is that enough for a chapter?"
"It doesn't matter, Rachel. A chapter can be as long or as short as you want it to be. It really doesn't matter."
"You gonna type everything I wrote?"
"Yes, I will, honestly!"
"Will you do it *all* today?"
"Okay."
"Will they tell you to rip it up?"
"Probably."
"But you won't, will you?"
"No."

CHAPTER FOUR   EXORCISM

"Jesus the name high over all,
In earth and heaven and sky.
Angels and men before it fall
And devils fear and fly!"

And *I* was supposed to fear and fly! I feared but I did not fly because I am not a demon. I am me. Rachel. I am Rachel. That is the first verse of a hymn they used to sing to me, four of them pinning Janet to the floor, and when they got to the last line about devils fearing and flying they would sing it extra loud and stare at me with nasty faces.

I was bloody terrified and I would scream blue murder and struggle till I was hot and sweaty and my head would feel like it was about to burst. Janet would cough and choke and retch and often she wet herself and a few times she stopped breathing and they had to shake her and push her tummy in and out until she started to breathe properly. Once Frankie had to put his mouth over hers and breathe into her because she went a funny colour and was not taking any breaths. Then she coughed and was sick and started to breathe again.

Exorcism means driving out demons and because I was a voice in Janet's head, then I was supposed to be a demon that had to be got rid of. For just over two years there were a lot of exorcisms. More than one a week sometimes. All the time we were getting worse. The Rev said that was because Satan was fighting stronger as the exorcisms progressed. What a load of s**t! I think now that Satan was laughing his bloody head off!!

THE HUDDLE

The sessions lasted from one hour up to eight hours, when they would bring Janet home at four or five in the morning.

It is the 19th February today and I am not feeling too good but I am trying to write this chapter all calm and sensible but I am not feeling like that because it is all very bad at the moment. Janet has got depression very bad and does not speak and she does not want me at all and after promising to type my writing up she broke her promise, and guess what she did last week? I had written seven and a half pages of this chapter and she ripped them all up and burned them in the kitchen sink because she saw the worms in the typewriter again, but then, that was not *my* fault, was it! She did not have to destroy *my* stuff, did she! I hate her. I was very upset and angry and I thought I was going to explode all over the place.

Then when Elinor came a few days ago on Monday she was nasty to me as well just because I got upset. She called it being firm, but I call it being NASTY! I chucked a few things and screamed a bit and got told off and to stop it at once and calm down and then she said that it was about time I let the Rev go out of my head and she wasn't going to put up with this sort of tantrum like I had with the Rev. Nasty, cruel cow! It was nothing like I was with the Rev. I hated him but I like her. I didn't swear at her or attack her and it didn't go on for hours and hours and it was the only time I have ever got like that in front of her in all the time I have known her! I lost my temper. I could not help it and she can go and whistle bloody Dixie!! (What the hell does 'whistle Dixie' mean? Who's this Dixie?)

And that is cruel. <u>F**KING</u> cruel! Telling me it's about time I let the Rev go! She's round the bloody twist. It's the other way around, about time <u>he</u> let <u>me</u> go!!! I have tried to get the Rev out of my head, I have screamed at him to go, and screamed at him to leave me alone, but he just shouts back at me, telling <u>me</u> to go. I can't get rid of him and he can't get rid of me. I do not want him in my head. I have asked Jesus nearly every day to take the Rev and the other bad voices away. I hate the Rev and I do not want him.

<u>I DO NOT WANT HIM IN MY HEAD!</u>
<u>I DO NOT WANT HIM IN MY HEAD!!</u>

<u>I DO NOT WANT HIM IN MY HEAD!!!</u>
<u>I DO NOT DELIBERATELY KEEP HIM IN MY HEAD!!!!</u>
<u>SILLY, NASTY CRUEL COW!!!!!</u>
<u>NASTY!!</u>

If I could just let him go then he would not be here, he would have gone ages ago and then I would not have some stupid, sodding bloody woman saying all this cruel f**king rubbish to me! If Jesus does not get the rev out of my head then how does the silly cow think I can do it? Cruel, nasty cow! Good job she is not a normal doctor, she would go around saying things like,
"I think it's about time you let go of your broken leg!
I think it's about time you should not have a heart attack!
I don't think you should hang on to your diabetes!"

HA! HA! HA!

THE HUDDLE

I had to do a lot of pretending with the Rev. I had to pretend I was a demon, pretend to go to the pit, pretend to be gone, and then pretend to be other demons because he would just keep on and on until he thought that the others that were supposed to be there were gone too. The exorcisms happened here at home, at the manse and in the church. Mostly they were at the manse.

A typical session might go something like this –

Janet would be frightened and hearing voices very loudly so they had to hold on to her as we got out of the car and drag her through the front door and into their living-room. It was not a nice living room and looked dingy and dusty and in the winter it was very cold and there was a hole in the carpet and they had put a chair over it to try and hide it. I saw it though. As soon as Janet sat down the voices and me would start yelling at her to get out. They would say,

"Look at the door, look at the door, get through it, get through it, get out of here, they're going to hurt you, look at the door, get out...."

Janet would turn her head to look at the door and the Rev and his wife, who looked like a vulture, would tell her not to listen to them but to resist them and listen to the Rev instead.

"Resist them in the name of the Lord! Resist the devil and he will flee from you!" (But he doesn't, does he!?)

There would be the Rev and his vulture wife, who talked too much, and usually an elder and his wife there as well. Janet was always made to sit on the same chair and the four of them would sit near her. The Rev would begin by committing the session to God and then he would read a passage out of the Bible. Something like about Jesus casting out demons, or about the resurrection, or from revelation all about Satan and the lake of fire and brimstone. Anything that would stir up the voices. Then he would pray and ask God to make any demons present manifest themselves, confess that Jesus is Lord, and go to the pit. That outer place of darkness. He would call down the wrath of God on all us voices and pray for us to be consigned forever to the everlasting darkness, eternal torment and the lake of fire and brimstone, Gehenna and Hell, the place reserved for Satan and his angels.

By this time Janet would be confused and terrified and get up to go but they would grab her and as she struggled they would pin her down either in the chair or on the floor. They even used to sit on her and that would drive her wild.

Then they would keep on and on and on.

"Who are you? Give me your name! I command you in the name of the Lord Jesus Christ, GIVE ME YOUR NAME and the names of the others that are with you!"

See, demons come in groups of three or seven. Three in imitation of the Trinity and seven to imitate God's number which is a bit up from the devil's 666. In each group there will be one leader spirit or 'master' who is in charge and stronger than the others in the group. This one will be the hardest to get rid of them and if you can get rid of him first then the others will quickly follow.

There were lots of groups of voices like this who went, but then others replaced them, so we were never without our voices. And many of us, us here

THE HUDDLE

now, we are not demons. But it was hopeless telling the Rev that we were not demons so in the end I used to make up some names. Sometimes he believed the names and sometimes he didn't. If he did believe the name he would say, like,

"Demon calling itself fear, I command you in the name of God, confess that Jesus is Lord! NOW! SAY IT! JESUS IS LORD!!!"

So I would pretend that I was this demon and say that Jesus is Lord and then he would say,

"Now go! OUT!! In the name of Jesus! Careeba de Gehenna bar yerkus ornam gemma ….. GO! Go to the pit!!"

Then the four of all at the same time would be telling me to go and I would be absolutely terrified and scream and struggle to get away from them. Maybe the elder and his wife would sing a hymn while the Rev and his wife kept on at me to get out and go. When I got too knackered to struggle any more, I would give up and go all quiet and limp, waiting for them to let go of me so that I could run. But then they took that to mean that the demon had gone and they would move on to the next demon and I would have to go through it all again. Lots of agains. Often I could not stick it for long and Janet would come back for a bit and she would beg them to take her home.

"Please take me home – I'm not a demon."

"Who are you?"

"Janet."

"You're not Janet! We know Janet. Now give me your name!"

"Janet."

"Oh no! The name by which you are known in hell!!"

Then they might just ignore her and start to sing loud hymns and she would get so upset that her arms and legs would start to twitch and her head went funny. She bit her tongue and wet her knickers lots of times.

In one of these sessions, if demons did not appear or would not go, then the Rev and his side kicks would ask Janet what unconfessed sin she was hiding that was preventing her being delivered.

"What hinders, Janet? What have you done? We know you've done something, come on, out with it!"

She used to go all dumb and stupid and I would tell her inside her head to make something up just to keep the Rev happy. So we told lies but we have told Elinor all about that and now it is alright. He seemed happier if Janet had done bad things all the time. And she did do bad things, but not all the time.

But thinking back a bit now, the Rev was really stupid because he did not seem to realise that a demon would never, ever confess that Jesus is Lord. A demon would be unable to do that and that is one of the things now that tell me I am not a demon. I can confess that Jesus is Lord. Angel tells me too that I am not a demon. Jesus is my friend and I like Him lots and I think that I love Him very much but sometimes I'm not sure and I get all these doubts and silly fears that are not silly when you are having them.

THE HUDDLE

So the Rev, he is pretty stupid for a Reverend. He does not know much about evil spirits and he does not know Jesus or angels either. Nasty, fat git!

Another thing he used to say to me that I now can't get out of my head is that,

"We hate you! God hates you! The whole of heaven hates you!!"

He told me that I had no right to be in Janet. I did not belong. I was evil and wicked and against God. But I *do* have a right to be here! This is *me*! Janet would not be able to be her if she did not have me. As we are plural then we can have a more special closeness to the state of being in Christ. Many in one is not of this world – it is closer to heaven and that is why we have got an angel in our head and I have Jesus in mine.

The Rev said all the time that Janet had to be delivered and that meant not hearing voices. So these exorcisms went on and on and on with us all getting worse and worse and worse. Terror! I was in terror! I got terrified of him. Once he called me a beast like the beast in the book of Revelation. He said he had got rid of hundreds of demons and that I would be got rid of in God's time. The demons had terrible, awful names… 20th April 1990.

("Rachel? Can I please not type all these down? Trying to forget! It's not good, let's not have all this putrid junk, *please*?"
"Okay. PIG!!")

Sometimes I thought the Rev wanted to screw with me so I would try to get him to do it so that it would be over with and then he would leave me alone. He shouted at me and called me a filthy beast.

Once when the voices were really bad, me and Janet couldn't cope with any more of all this crap and so the Rev ended up taking Katy to the manse. Katy used to be blind because of the dogs and the Rev thought she was Janet under the influence of a demon of blindness or sightlessness. When they got Katy out of the car at the manse they didn't tell her about the step by the front door and she tripped and started to cry. They told her to go to hell as well. They told all of us to go there. And Janny. She got shouted at because she would not speak anything. I think she was too frightened.

At the end of any of these sessions, the Rev might have to spend ages calling Janet back. Sometimes it did not work and even I do not know who he brought home and who Frankie had to put to bed. Frankie had to stay home and look after Janet and the kidlets and he nearly lost his job and they had no money coming in and the Rev said that it was Janet's fault they had no money because she was not co-operating and was not able to hold down a job. Balls to all that mate! Six weeks after the second time we were in St. Cadoc's, Janet went and got a job and he was gobsmacked! Then he was afraid that I would cause trouble for her in work and things were really bad. Pig of a man!

The voices never went away and I used to beg Janet not to see the Rev any more and then she used to beg Frankie not to make her see him but he said that if she didn't then they would not have a marriage and the Rev said he had grounds for a divorce and that Janet would not get custody of her

THE HUDDLE

kids because she was an unfit mother because of the voices and cutting herself and being in St. Cadoc's.

When Janet got anorexic the Rev and Mrs. Rev said she had a demon called 'Anorexia' and they tried to get rid of it but it didn't work and Janet kept getting lighter. Once they forced her to eat a welsh cake. They said she couldn't go home until she ate it and the tears were coming out fast as she forced it down her throat. She was sick on the way home.

Sometimes during these exorcism sessions they would sprinkle her with water because demons don't like water. They lit a fire a few times as well and told us that was like the fires of hell where we were going, only hell was much worse. I was very frightened of their fire and they made Janet burn lots of her writing and music in this fire because they said it had been written under the influence of demons.

Often we were not offered a drink for hours and hours and we would be hot and sweaty from struggling on the floor with four people. Janet would ask for a drink and get a drop of water in a plastic cup thing which they used to keep hold of while she drank.

They said she was not safe to be with her kids. They were worried about the kids because they said that Janet was possessed by a demon called Molech, who used to burn children on altars and there were also demons like paedophilia and perversion and rape and infanticide. They all wanted to do bad things to the chickadees according to the Rev. Frankie has just read this paragraph and he says that it is true. That is what the Rev said.

It did not take long before I started acting like a demon every time I saw the bloody Rev! When I was *not* a demon he still shouted at me and called me evil and said he hated me and God hated me and the whole of heaven hated me, so I thought, right!! If I am going to always be treated like a bloody demon then I might as well always *act* like a bloody demon!

It was easy to swear and say bad things when I was so angry and upset and scared. I was told I was an abomination, obscene, stinking, evil, wicked, foul, filthy, a fiend, Satan's servant, I disgusted the Rev, I was useless, not wanted, and lots and lots more. It went on and on and on and in the end I remember really, really believing that I was an evil spirit because I came to feel that I was everything he was saying about me.

It took Elinor ages to convince me I was not a demon. I think that mostly I believe her now but there is still an incey wincey bit of me that wonders if I am a demon and it is just a trick of Satan that now leads me to believe that I am not. You see, well, I have to share a body and that is not easy and I get awful thoughts in my head and very often I wish I *was* a demon and I could be got rid of and then I would not be here. It must be better for us all to be dead but Angel says we must not do it.

Frankie is home looking after us both today because Janet is very depressed and we both want, me and Janet that is, to kill ourselves more than we want anything else. I do not think I can

THE HUDDLE

hang on much longer and I don't think Janet can either. It does not matter.

The Rev had a 'thing' about blood and used to go on a lot about Janet needing to be washed and cleansed in the blood of Christ. It reminded us of having blood on us in witchcraft and we thought it was revolting for Christians to be washed in blood. They used to sing this hymn to us. I will write down the first verse.

"There is a fountain filled with blood
Drawn from Immanuel's veins.
And sinners plunged beneath that flood
Lose all their guilty stains."

Me and the voices used to go mad! Me and Janet still hate that hymn. It makes us feel sick! Then he was always on about hell and death and destruction and the second death and repentance and forgiveness. A few times I prayed out loud for Jesus to forgive me and save me from all this Gehenna and everlasting torment but then the Rev would laugh and tell me that there was no mercy for demons and God would not help me.

I hate the Reverend! HATE HIM! GET OUT OF MY BLOODY HEAD!!!! PIG! PIG!! PIG!!! <u>PIG!!!!</u>   I can't shout loud enough on paper.

He would call down the wrath of God on me and tell me that the longer I resisted going to hell then the worse my punishment would be when I eventually got there to where I belonged. The place reserved for me and my kind. Everlasting chains of darkness and eternal damnation. No fellowship in hell. No love. Only the torment I so richly deserved.

"Why are you doing this to me?" I would always ask the Rev and his wife.

"Because we hate you and we love Janet. Now GO! OUT!! In the name of Jesus!"

"NO! I'm not going, I won't go, I live here!"

"O yes you will go! My God says you will go! I am a servant of the living God and by the power invested in me I now command you to leave this woman!"

Me and Janet would be brought home from these Exorcisms exhausted, dishevelled, bruised, scratched, face swollen from crying and screaming, sore, and aching all over. It was very, very bad and I do not think I am very good at describing just how bad it was but I am having a go

I tried to tell the Rev that Jesus loved me. He did not believe me and he laughed and said I was deluded by my own master, Satan.

"Who is your master?" He would ask me and he was being sarcastic.

"Jesus!"

"Oh no! You are one of Satan's little minions! Satan is *your* master!"

The Rev was making fun of me so bit by bit I acted more and more like a demon and I got to be really good at it. Then I believed that I was one. I made Janet worship Satan with me and we did spells against the Rev so that he would leave us alone and not be able to hurt us. God did not stop him from hurting us and so we asked the devil instead. Then the Rev would find out what Janet had been up to and force her to pray for forgiveness, pray to renounce the devil and all his works, and to be cleansed in the blood of Christ

THE HUDDLE

and be completely delivered. When she could not speak any words he would say she had a dumb spirit, a spirit of prayerlessness or a spirit of rebellion.

"How dare you not obey God, Janet? How *dare* you!! God commands all men everywhere to repent. NOW PRAY!"

Once Janet had conjunctivitis and the Rev prayed that the sin or the demon causing it would be dealt with by God. But then Dr. Sami sent her to St. Woolos and they put needles in and washed out her tear ducts, so it was not demons or sin. It was blocked tear ducts. But the Rev still thought they were blocked by sin and demons.

Janet and me was made a scapegoat for things that were not right in his church and he said that when me and all the other voices went then God would bless his church.

His exorcisms were a load of bloody crap and if I could get all this s**t out of my head, then I would. Elinor is nasty to imply that I can when I can't Don't like that. I have tried to get rid of it all. I don't want it. I hate it. It won't go. The Rev won't get out of my head. She's the bloody psychiatrist, so why doesn't she get him out of my head? She does not understand and I thought she did. I feel like hurting her now but I still want a big hug off her and I do not understand why I feel so mixed up. She is supposed to unmix me! I am all mixed up and horrible and I know it must be my fault.

Then the Rev would make me open my eyes and look up to heaven because he said that if I did then I would have to go to hell because I could not bear the glory I would see. He would say,

"Look! Look! You can't look, can you! Now go! Leave this woman. Do not harm her as you go and go to the pit. NOW! GO! I command you in the name of the Lord Jesus Christ, GO!!"

Lots of times the Rev would make Janet feel awful by telling her that they had had nothing to eat all day because of having to deal with her in the evening. 'This sort goeth out by nothing but prayer and fasting.' Or something like that. It is in the Bible somewhere. So she would be made to feel terrible and guilty.

It never seemed to end and it never seems to end. Often I feel as if it is happening to me all over again and I curl up in my cell and scream my head off for hours and hours and hours. Janet hates me doing that, it drives her nuts. Don't care! Or I lie down and thrash about and scream and fight him off.

It has been very bad for me to be told all those things that the Rev told me. Me and Janet, we both find it very difficult and very hurting to read certain parts of the Bible and sing certain hymns. It reminds us, and feels like it is all thrashing through our head again. Sometimes very fast and sometimes in slow motion. We hear the Rev's voice and smell the manse and feel his grip on our wrists.

I think that this sort of exorcism is dangerous and should not be done to people. Jesus did not do this sort of thing. It is very cruel. Witches are still human beings and Jesus still loves them just as much as He loves the Christians, even though he really hates what witches get up to. I do not think anyone should dare to tell someone else that God hates them. It is serious. Very bad. Exorcism is

THE HUDDLE

very bad. I wish it had not happened. It got Janet really hating me and me really hating her and we never really have been friends or got on okay since. She became convinced I was a demon as well and has tried to exorcise herself to get rid of me and the others. That was very scary and it made the voices worse.

I am in a mess. I do not know how to get out of it and mostly I do not want to be here. I want to go to heaven because I know that when I see Jesus I will be okay. Exorcism made me hate Jesus and turn my back on Him but now I am friends with Him again and I think that the Rev must know a different Jesus to the one I love. My Jesus is not cruel and does not want to get rid of me. Exorcism nearly took Him away from me. Exorcism is bad.

Exorcism - was forcing something on us that we didn't want. Janet said the Rev should have told her to go to her doctor, but he didn't, he kept saying the doctors and psychiatrists would not help her.

Exorcism - meant telling her to go to the manse against her will and not letting her go home when she wanted to. It meant reading lots of the Bible *against* us and saying lots of prayers *against* us and singing lots of hymns *against* us and against me to frighten me away.

Exorcism – was saying that they hated me and God hated me and wanted to drive me into hell and it was always the telling of me to go and get out and that I was unwanted. Janet does not want me now.

Exorcism – was the servant of God doing what God told him to do. It still goes round inside out head like lots of mad bad flashes and echoes.

Exorcism – was holding us down by force and frightening us stupid. It sent us mad and we had to go to hospital.

When they held her on the floor at the manse her clothes went all over the place and then when they tried to take blood off her in the hospital she went nuts and they had to hold her down until she got quiet and calm again.

Exorcism hurt us and scared us and made us hate God and the church and Christians and made us want to be dead all the time and it made us frightened of Bibles and we used to rip them up and do bad things with the pages and we are both still very frightened of God. We have been going to another church for a few weeks and that frightens us but Janet has to go because one of the chickadees sings in the choir and is very good at it. I am very terrified of being in this church and I don't know what will happen. Don't want to write or think or talk about it. I am scared and I don't want to go there and I don't want to be here.

I have just asked her and Janet says,

"My exorcism was abusive, intrusive, offensive, humiliating, faith shattering, inducive of suicidal tendencies, severely depressing, emotionally damaging, soul destroying, spiritually shattering and, worst of all, probably totally unnecessary!"

I've got Janet angry and upset again now by asking her about that. She does not like me at all. She said we should have had gentle services of deliverance and not these full scale exorcisms, but I am not sure I understand the difference between exorcism and deliverance.

THE HUDDLE

In the Bible when Jesus did exorcisms He never did what the Rev and his hangers on did to us. He was not cruel and He did not shout. The Rev took Jesus away from me and he should not have done that and it is a wonder I have started to believe in Him again but hearing His voice and having an angel in my head helps a bit. They both tell me that I won't go to hell like the Rev keeps telling me, but they don't shut him up and get rid of him and I don't know why not because I know that they both like me and love me. Elinor says she loves me but she was still nasty to me on Monday when I lost my temper a bit.

There is a verse somewhere in the Bible about the Rev and what he did to me and Katy and Janny. I do not know if he did it to the others as well. This verse says that whoever offends a little one that believes in Jesus, it would be better for that person if a stone was hung around his neck and he was thrown into the sea! So there!! I've got nothing else to say now that I have said that about him!

I think that if I had a really good think and tried hard then I could remember lots more bad stuff about the exorcisms but I have only written down the bits that are easily in my head all the time without having to stop and think. Angel has said not to try and remember any more because that would not be good for me. So I won't. She says that it is good for me to have forgotten lots of it and I must never try to drag things up.

I wish the Rev would get out of my head. He does not look very nice and he does not say nice things. I wish he would go away for ever and I wish that the exorcisms had never happened.

The end of this chapter.

THE HUDDLE

CHAPTER FIVE   MY JESUS

"My Jesus I love Thee, I know Thou art mine;
For Thee all the pleasures of sin I resign;
My gracious Redeemer, my Saviour art Thou,
If ever I loved Thee, my Jesus, 'tis now."

And I do love Him and I've given up lots of bad sins that were nice at the time and I am trying to give up a few more as well. I think that I must be still very wrong and bad and full of sin.

Do you know what Janet once yelled at me? That I was 'surplus to her requirements!' – A bit of surplus? That means a bit of something that is not necessary and it is not a very nice thing to say and I felt very upset and horrible inside and like a bit of unwanted rubbish that should be chucked in the bin. Made me feel like a right load of tat, that did. (What is tat?)

Jesus inside my head says that nobody is surplus, not even me, and everyone here in this head is equally special even if we feel like a bunch of misfits.

Janet says that she feels like the host to a group of parasites, but I am not a parasite, I am Rachel and we that are here are not parasites. Jesus loves all of us the same, even if some of us don't love Him just yet, and that sort of loving can be hard to take in because I want Him to love me more than he loves the others. But then, seeing as there are a few of us here, we must have an awful lot of Jesus available to us because if He has got a chunk of love for me and one for Jan and chunks for Janet and Liz and Katy and Janny and I know there are another two, then for one body, that adds up to a very much lot of love. So therefore we are very, very much greatly loved, all rolled into one, so if we all loved Him back the same, there would be oodles of love pouring out of an us all together.

I think that Jesus is the most special to me. He loved me when we were a witch and did bad things and I don't know what I am now but I know that He loves me just as much because He tells me deep inside myself. I do not know much *about* Jesus because I do not read the Bible hardly at all and the Rev really put me off Him for ages, but I do *know* Jesus and I think that is more important than knowing all about His life and the miracles and parables and things. My Jesus seems like a different Jesus from the one the rev was on about. My Jesus loves me.

The thing is, I do not ever want to be called a Christian because, if you ask me, there are some bloody funny Christians about and I don't want to be like them and I don't want to be called the same as the Rev who calls himself a Christian. So I have just had a thought that I could call me a 'Jesus Person' instead and that will simply mean that I have Jesus inside me and I love Him and I like him. I think that might be a good thing to call me. I am Rachel and I am a Jesus Person. I like that.

Me is like Janet in that I can't get on with all this God, and Father God, and loving heavenly Father bit. I can't work it out and I don't like it and so for twits like us who don't like the God bit, there came Jesus. I never do think much about Jesus being the Son of God but I do know that the Bible says that He is. The Bible also says that of you know Jesus

THE HUDDLE

then you also know His Father, so I don't *have* to get to grips with this God stuff, do I! I have Jesus and that is enough, because God is too big and He punishes people and allows illness and hurting and lots of bad things like the devil and murder and raping and hurting kids. He even watched Jesus being hammered onto a cross by people that He had made and loved. I do not understand Him and I do not want to know Him.

God did not help any of us when very bad things were happening. He watched and he did nothing and He let it happen. Jesus watched as well and He wanted to come and help us but He couldn't because He was pinned to a cross and he couldn't get down from it and He was hurting as much as we were, and more, because He was made to watch but not able to save us from it. I think that must have been very awful for Him because he loves us so much. He did not want the bad to happen either, and He cried a lot. He cried for everybody's bad bits and He understands and if you talk to Him then He will listen and know what you are on about and how bad you feel because He has felt very bad as well. He understood on Monday when I lost my temper, but He didn't get his hair off like Elinor did. I think she had better spend more time talking to Him!

So I will forget the Son of God bit. Can't manage that. Jesus is just Jesus. That is enough and that is everything. I call Him that! Jesus. I don't call Him 'the Lord', or 'Christ', or 'Jesus Christ', or 'the Lord Jesus Christ' because all of them don't sound very friendly and can sound like you are swearing. He is Jesus!

Also, I do not think of Jesus as being a man because He does not have thoughts about me like a man could have, and I am very glad about that because it is one of the best things about Him. He does not want me for sex; He wants me just because I am me. I know that Jesus *was* a man when He was on earth but now that He is in heaven He is different and back to normal and so therefore He is far more special than just being a man.

I hate men. Men are stupid and nasty. When I speak and I write about Jesus, I say 'Him' and 'His' and 'He', but He is *not* a man to me, or for me, or towards me. He is Jesus. I do not see Him now having the body of a man. He is Jesus. My Jesus!

I think about some very pretty flowers and lots and lots of different colours; like roses and fuscias and crocuses and wallflowers and pansies. They are very lovely and if you could roll up their colours and loveliness into one, then that would be almost as lovely as Jesus is. He can be a snowdrop, very white and pure and delicate, and yet still a snowdrop can push up and out of the hard and frosty ground. Like Jesus trying to get through to Janet. He is very gentle and she is hard and frosty. The snowdrop always wins the fight and gets through in the end.

Or Jesus can be a gladiolus! Very strong, sturdy and upright, easy to see and to like and to admire. When He is a host of golden daffodils there is too much of Him and I love Him too much and I don't know what to do about it. I think I should pick bunches of Him and give then to people, like people who hear voices, or who are sad, or who

THE HUDDLE

are being raped. Jesus is masses of the most prettiest colours.

He is a smell much better than Lyle's Golden syrup, of Freesias, or toast when you are hungry. Sweet and lovely and nice so that you want more and more and more of Him. Jesus is lots of tinkly bluebells on a summer's day. He is drifts of pink and white blossom, he is strong, purple Heather, He is an oak tree, He is velvety green grass and He is dew on a spider's web that twinkles like lots of diamonds when the sun shines on it. He is so many colours, and then some more, and the colours are very beautiful. He is very beautiful. Jesus. My Jesus.

Jesus is a warm and a bright light that lives right down the very middle of me, like the core in an apple, and the apple would not live and grow without its core. I know that. Even though I might not be able to see this bright light, I know that it is there. It is brilliant and it would dazzle me and I would have to close my eyes tight. I will be able to see it when I am in heaven. That is something to look forward to. Angel says that I have to live and so I try to keep thinking that however bad life is, then at least I have something to look forward to at the end of it. Like a reward for staying here and putting up with things. My reward, that I shall see Jesus in heaven and he will make us all better and we will be all okay. There will not be the bad voices in heaven; it is a lot of things to look forward to.

Janet can't pray with words and I don't either really, though I do have one prayer that I say over and over again a lot. I think it is called the 'Jesus

Prayer' and Elinor wrote it down on a piece of paper for us ages ago. I say it like this,

"Jesus have mercy on me, a sinner." Sometimes I just say 'Jesus'. It is a very good name to say when my voices are bad and I think I am going nuts, and I say it as well in any odd sorts of moments when I happen to remember about it.

Janet says, who the hec do I think I am? One of those nuns who lock themselves away in a cell and pray the same thing over and over again? I say to her, well, what is wrong with that? Sometimes when I say this prayer Jesus gives me a cuddle. It is not like this body being given a hug by another human being. It is a very special cuddle and feels like the very most important bit of me is extra loved and extra safe and extra precious. It feels like me and Jesus are all rolled into one and I do this deep groaning into Him that feels nicer inside than anything I have ever felt. For a few seconds it feels as if the world and Janet and all the bad has gone away and all that matters is being in Jesus and Him in me and being so safe and lovely and clean. That is a Jesus hug.

I can talk to Jesus without using any words and He can understand me.

("You mean you can communicate with Him without speaking!"
"Get lost! This is ME writing and you are not to say ANYTHING, so sod off!)

I MEAN THAT I CAN TALK TO JESUS WITHOUT SAYING ANY WORDS! And He understands me.

THE HUDDLE

When I ask Him things He does not always answer me how I want him to. I keep asking Him why He does not take away the bad voices and all that happens for a reply is that Angel says to trust Him. Maybe He feels bad about me having the voices and so gets someone else to speak for Him. I don't get it.

I do not understand about the Holy Spirit or the Holy Ghost. Spirits and ghosts are devils and demons and they are evil and Jesus cannot be with anything that is evil because He has never done anything wrong or evil and He never will do. Is the Holy Spirit or Ghost really an angel? Angels are good spirits from heaven so they must be holy and so an angel must be a holy spirit. If so, then I have a holy spirit in me and it says that people who love Jesus have to be filled with this spirit. So am I alright because we have angel?

Today is a day that I don't feel able to talk to Jesus because all my wrong and bad spilled out on Monday and I feel like hiding myself away for ever and being dead. So I will just have to say my Jesus prayer instead.

I think that the most amazing thing about Jesus is that he loves me. It is very hard to love me because I am not very nice although I do not swear as badly as I used to when I was a demon. But I have done some very awful things. I used to shout very loud, in very bad language, saying that I hated Jesus. I have prayed to Satan and done spells and called up evil spirits and Jesus hates witchcraft. I am nasty to Janet and the others and I do not even feel sorry about it. But He still loves me. When He died on the cross it was so that all my bad bits would not matter any more. Like God punishing Him for them instead of punishing me. The Rev called it…

(What did he call it?
"Substitutional atonement."
Ta!)

The Rev called it that. So my bad bits don't matter to Jesus, but I still feel very terrible about them; all guilty and embarrassed. Angel says I don't *need* to feel like this but I still do. I am very stupid and all wrong and mixed up inside. But Jesus still loves me. The only other person who says they love me is Elinor but I think she has to say that because she is a doctor and she is supposed to make me feel better about myself. She wears these millions of big rings and always has half a pair of glasses hanging around her neck. Jesus loves Elinor as well. She must be easier to love than I am except when she is ratty and in a bad mood.

Jesus is not like human beings. He does not get bad moods or lose His temper or shout or get nasty with me. He is always the same. He is gentle and strong and calm and quiet and safe. It is very safe to love Jesus because He is not capable of hurting me and He would never want to. I know that. He is *worth* loving and I am not a disappointment to Him because He loves me exactly as I am. Me! Rachel! Even if I never got better then He would still love me just the same.

I don't think I can write any more now. I am tired and I want to go away to nowhere. I hope I have written properly about Jesus.

THE HUDDLE

He will never ever leave me and he is my Jesus for ever.
> To Jesus,
> Luv Rachel.

The voices hate Jesus and are always saying very, very bad things to me about him. They keep telling me that He does not love me and that He will do bad things to me but I mostly am able to remember that they are all liars.

They also tell me that Jesus is Satan in disguise and Satan is playing tricks on me and all of us here. The voices would like to kill Jesus and know that He was dead. Sometimes I can think that the voices are frightened of Him because they never actually get around to doing any of the bad things to Him that they talk about doing.

I think that because I am now a Jesus Person then the bad voices are trespassers onto holy ground and that is very dangerous for them. They are jealous of Jesus because He is Jesus and they are not and I love Jesus but I do not love them. I hate them very much. My Jesus could get rid of the voices if He wanted to. I do not know why He doesn't.

The best thing about being in heaven will be seeing Jesus as He really is. The Bible says there are no tears in heaven so therefore there can not be bad voices either because bad voices make you cry. Jesus is going to wipe away all my tears with a great big Kleenex when I am in heaven and then I will be better for ever.

A big AMEN!

Janet Cooper

THE HUDDLE

CHAPTER SIX   A LETTER TO THE VOICES

Me. Rachel. I am going to try and write this without swearing too much. I do not want to sound like them but it is difficult to get angry on paper without putting in the swear words and when I write about the voices I do get to feel angry.

To the bad voices,
Sometimes I call you <u>my</u> voices instead of <u>the</u> voices or <u>bad</u> voices and I am trying hard not to call you my voices because you are *not* mine! And I am not yours! I do not want you or own you and I never asked you to come here and stick around with me. So you are *not* mine!!

You are all very bad and very rotten and you stink, the worst smell we've ever smelled. We keep a perfume stick by us all the time so we can sniff it and get away from your awful stink. You are a bad smell in our nose like decay and sick and bad eggs and gone off milk and bad s**t all rolled into one and stewed in the hot sun. You are sometimes like a bad taste in our mouth as if we are sucking dirty pennies. Evil metal, you are!

You are Satan's mad chatterbox.
Bats.
You are batty and you are bats.
Lots of black bats.
Battering bats.
Splattering bats.

You are the bats from hell that batter my ears and splatter dirty words all over my thinking; black bats that keep coming at me, flapping around me and fluttering in my face so that all there seems to be of life are you. Swooping and threatening. I dodge to get out of your way but I can't.

Even when I cannot hear you I know what you are saying. Why don't you leave me alone? Why do you only say rude and bad and nasty things? Who sent you to me? Who *are* you? Why have *I* got to hear you? If you hate me so much then why don't you go away?

You have invaded my head and my cell and you are trespassers and you are so ugly that I can't think up the words to describe you. I bet Janet could. I do not want you. I do not want to hear bad voices all the time. Don't you ever go to sleep?

You make me so angry and then I want to scream and do bad things. Very sometimes you make me strong and I fight against you and against the bad that you are always on about. Mostly you make me sad and frightened and I put my hands over my ears or my arms around my head, trying to shut you out of me and away from me. And then all you do is laugh at me.

You are my tormentors and my bullies and my enemies. *Have* you come to punish me for the bad that I did? Wasn't Jesus punished enough? YES! HE WAS!!! So you should not be here. Yet you have always been here. Why?

Then you make me feel so fed up and fat and ugly and freaky and dirty that I cry. Then you laugh some more. I do not think I could be more hated than I am by you lot. I hate *you* too! You make me

THE HUDDLE

feel like s**tty rubbish that should be kicked out of sight. Like I am too bad to be here and I should be dead. You tell me all the time to kill myself, and then I want to. So then you laugh some more.

You make me very unhappy and nobody can know about me or like me. You make it so hard for me not to swear, and hard for me to be nice, and hard for me to love Jesus properly; you just make everything so very. Very hard. You make me feel like I am in the middle of a war and I am never going to win; as if I have to keep on fighting but I'll never get anywhere. You are a very strong and a very cruel enemy.

You are beetles on the wall, in the chair and in the pillow. You are all the worms in the typewriter. You are the maggots in a bowl of porridge. You are the fear and the being scared all the time. You make me feel as if I do not know what I am thinking and can't remember what I have just said. You make everything so difficult and there is no being happy while I have you. You make me very miserable. You are the reason why I do not want to live.

Do you want to know something else? You won't like it! You are also the reason why Jesus is so nice and so lovely and so wonderful for me. Because you are so bad, the comparison with Him is so enormous that I love Him more. Yes, I do, because I have you lot! I can see how He is opposite to you. He is everything good and you are not. He has brought some light and you make me feel dark, like black lumps of shiny coal. He is heaven and you are hell. I choose heaven. I choose Jesus.

Janet Cooper

I am closer to Jesus because of you because you frighten me into Him. Because you are so bad I have to snuggle up to Him, closer and closer to try and get away from you. I pray my Jesus prayer lots more when you are especially loud and cruel to me. So you really do make me pray more and love Jesus more. This is a funny way of looking at it. Have I written it down properly, what I mean to say? Have I?

("Yes, Rachel, you're okay, carry on."
You nice to me now after Monday? I didn't mean to do all that.
"Just get on with this, will you? It doesn't matter about Monday – we'll sort it out.")

You make me feel that there is all this fighting inside me between light and dark and between Jesus and Satan and between all of you and me. A big war is going on inside me and around me and Satan wants me to be back on his side and there are times when I think it would be *easier* to belong to him and give in to all you bad things. Fighting makes me so tired all the time. Jesus wants me and Satan wants me and I am not worth all this wanting. It does not make any sense to me and I do not get it.

YOU, the bad voices, you keep me in hell. You are the clappers of hell that keep clanging at me. Noises of hell. Sounds of hell. Voices of hell. My cell is hell! That rhymes! I have a hell inside my cell. Voices that all the time are clanging at me and ringing in my ears and battering my brain. Voices? – You are pain and you hurt and you are hurting me

THE HUDDLE

and you are not doing me any good and you are very bad for me.

I would like you all to go away as soon as possible. I would like some quiet without you reminding me all the time of bad and nasty things and calling me names and hating me all the day long. I do not think I can put up with you much longer and then where will you go to when I am soon dead? I would like to scream and go nuts again now but Angel says that I do not need to do that. It is very hard to hear voices. I wish other people could hear them just so they could know what it was like and I wish that Elinor could hear them, but only for a very short bit, so that she would know what they are like as well. I am very sorry for me.

Are you the same voices that Janet hears? I would never ever call you a huddle because that sounds too friendly for pigs like you. If I was going to give you a name, and I'm bloody well *not* going to, then I would call you something like 'The Devil's Gang', or 'S**t People'. I would never call you anything nice.

I want you to listen to this prayer that I am saying to Jesus. I am not very good at prayers, but he doesn't mind that, as long as I try. I would say, 'Jesus, You know all about the voices and how bad they are and that I feel lonely and sad and horrible because of them. I think that you might know more about them than I do. I am trying very hard to believe that You are stronger than they are and that You are able to get the damn things off me. Jesus, please take all the bad voices away from me. I am so fed up and miserable and I can't stop thinking about going nuts or killing myself. They are driving me round the bloody twist! Please take them away. Please! From Rachel.'

I can hear you now, voices, telling me off because I swore in a prayer. *You* swear *all* the time! I think you are what they call a bunch of bloody hypocrites. What else do they say? 'You are enough to make a saint swear!'

One day I hope that you will be gone and then I will feel lots better and be a nice person and feel like I am clean. I hope that you rot in your own hell.
Yours sincerely,
Rachel.

Guess what? There is a hymn in Janet's hymn book that has the most *awful* tune to it, like Munster music, and Janet often reads this hymn and I have read it a lot with her. It reminds her of The Huddle and it reminds me of the voices that I hear. It has got four verses. I will write them down.

("Rachel, don't write all the verses out, tell me which hymn it is and I'll type it out for you."
Why can't I write the verses out?
"Because there's no point really, is there! I'll be typing all this out anyway; I can look it up in the hymn book."
But I *want* to write them down! It's *my* writing and *I* can do what the bloody hell I...
"Okay, okay! Have it your own way! Do what the hell you like!"
I *WILL*!!!!!!)

THE HUDDLE

The hymn goes like this. And I want to do *all* the verses!

Christian dost thou see them
On the holy ground,
How the powers of darkness
Compass thee around?
Christian, up and smite them,
Counting gain but loss;
For your mighty saviour
Triumphed on the cross.

Christian dost thou feel them,
How they work within?
Striving, tempting, luring,
Goading into sin?
Christian never tremble,
Never be downcast;
Gird thee for the conflict,
Watch and pray and fast.

Christian, dost thou hear them,
How they speak thee fair?
'Always fast and vigil?
Always watch and prayer?'
Christian answer boldly,
'While I breathe I pray';
Peace shall follow battle,
Night shall end in day.

'Well I know thy trouble,
O my servant true;
Thou art very weary –
I was weary too:

Janet Cooper

But that toil shall make thee
Some day all mine own,
And the end of sorrow
Shall be near my throne.'

My favourite verse is the last one because it is Jesus talking to me but He is saying that I won't really be happy until I am near His throne and to be near his throne means being in heaven.

Janet, she is very depressed today and has been sitting lots with the headphones on and then Janny sucked her thumb and kept knocking a little toy dog off the coffee table. Janny gets on my nerves and Janet does not want to be alive but she has been reading this hymn. I am only going to write the first verse this time.

Far off I see the goal;
O Saviour, guide me;
I feel my strength is small;
Be Thou beside me:
With vision ever clear,
With love than conquers fear,
And grace to persevere,
O Lord provide me.

To the voices – you have ruined our lives and you make us not want to be alive and living because everything is spoiled by you. Even if we look at a flower and think that it is pretty you will spoil it for us by saying the flower is f**king rubbish and should be covered in dog s**t. Then you would tell us to eat the s**t. You spoil everything and we got no friends or nice feelings or being happy

THE HUDDLE

because of you. You make Jesus so beautiful and perfect.
>To the voices,
>**WE HATE YOU!!!!!!**

CHAPTER SEVEN   MY FUTURE

It is lots of months later now and we should finish this book. We are both feeling better (Janet and me) but there has been some trouble with Katy and Elinor had to talk to her again but she is a lot better again now. So I will do a last chapter and Janet will do a very, very last chapter and tell what has happened to us and how it happened. It is very nice but very scary.

I still have my voices and I pray a lot. The Rev drives me nuts and he would not like it that we have joined a choir with a church with altars and candles and things. Janet said she will write about how we came to be in a church choir. It is lovely and I like it a lot and feel very close to Jesus because I wear lovely robes and sing to Him and I can hide in my robes and it is a big thing that Janet and I can do together because Angel said we were to do it together. I don't know if I could say that I am friends with Janet again yet, but it has helped a lot to do something together. We are not so sad and depressed now either.

The voices are very bad in church so I said I would take the bread and the wine bit for Janet because she found it too bad, but it was bad for me too and they kept telling me to spit out the wine and spill the chalice and much worse things than that. Then Janet and Elinor went to Monmouth to see a lady called Una who lives by a church and I didn't want to go because I was scared this lady would hate me and want to get rid of me, but then when we got there she was beautiful and gave me a very big and safe hug, and I hugged her back and told

THE HUDDLE

her that I liked her because I do. And she told us that if the bread and wine made the voices worse, that don't take it for a bit. That made church lots easier for us both.

Then about a week after that Elinor sent me a letter and told me that she didn't ever want me to go away and that made me feel better as well. I am not too much friends with Frankie at the moment but it isn't *too* bad and the worst bit is that we have someone else in this head called Hestia. Me and Janet tried to pretend for ages that she did not exist and Janet still thinks she is a Huddle voice, but last Monday she talked to Elinor and was very horrible so I would not listen and Janet would not listen either.

So now we are seven but maybe that is right because seven is God's number and we like things to go in sevens and threes. Hestia does not love Jesus like I do or like Janet wants to. I do not know if she has Angel. She is very bad and dark and nasty and I wish we did not have her, then last Friday, in the shower, her and Liz got together and cut Janet with a knife and Dr. Sami had to put stitches in the cuts and it is the first cuts we have had for nearly a year so Janet says that is not bad, but really she thinks it is very bad and we are very upset about it.

I feel frightened but Angel tells me to think about the disciples in the boat with Jesus, they were frightened in the storm but were safe because Jesus was always with them. I know that He is with me, it is hard to always believe, but I have Him in my very middle and I love Him more than anything.

I think that if God said so, then Jesus would get rid of my voices.

In the church in Monmouth I knelt on the floor in a little chapel thing where there were four angels up high and Elinor knelt by me too and I prayed to ask Jesus to make me better. Elinor said prayers too, but I do not know what she prayed about.

Me and Janet had a dream about Angel telling Elinor about us getting better. I would like to write it down, and the other dreams, but Hestia has been very nasty and she has ripped up our dream diary.

At the moment I have gone all quiet inside. I do feel very sad and upset and it would be better to already be in heaven, but tomorrow I will put on my lovely robes and sing to Jesus in a big and lovely place. I am not special, but I will feel special just for him and for just a little while, and then maybe the sun inside me will shine a little bit more. Now I am dull and sleepy. Last night Jesus put His hands around our crazy head and for a few seconds it was like a little bit of heaven. Janet says it was a dream. But it wasn't. It was really Him!

I still want to not have the voices and I would still prefer to be dead, but things *are* lots better for us and I know that I have to stay here, even when it is very hard, and I have to be okay.

I am still very good friends with Elinor even though a few weeks ago I lost my temper and broke a few things, but she didn't stop liking me, so it's alright again now. I call her my nice old bag! I do not know what I will do when she goes away but I can still write to her but it won't be the same because no-one will give me a hug and I think I will

THE HUDDLE

cry a bit about that. I don't know what will happen to me then.

So this is a last chapter to say that everything is a lot better, except for Hestia, and that I am mostly feeling lots better than I was. Janet says we will write another book one day and it will be a happy one instead of like this one, full of bad bits. But then, maybe if we hadn't written about the bad bits, and lived through the bad bits, then there could never *be* the happy bits!!

From,
Rachel.

Janet Cooper

A FEW MONTHS LATER   (By me, Janet!)

Now, many months after I wrote the last sentence of my book, and typed the last sentence of Rachel's book, I am amazed to be passing at least some of my time in an undepressed state. It is like a light being sometimes turned on for me, I realise just a little that I am a much loved and wanted part of a family, and I also know the pure joy of feeling happy and being able to smile.

I recognise that my life is one long unplanned journey. Some plans have not happened. For so long now I have planned *not* to be alive by teatime, tomorrow, next week or next month. I cannot in all honesty say yet that I am *glad* to be alive, because the brief glimpses of sunshine are so new. It is scary and there are still days when I am plunged back into deepest darkness and rotting, secretly, so secretly still longing for the release that my suicide would be for me. I am on a rollercoaster of agony and ecstasy and this is a confusing and perplexing time. It is also a time of love and healing, a time to be humble and patient, and a time to seek to become closer to God.

I still have The Huddle. In fact they are no different. What *is* different is the improvement in my depressed mood and therefore, consequently, an improvement in my ability to cope with their continual daily torment. I also find, these past weeks, that I am not gripped by so great a fear of them, and this loses them a little of their powerful hold upon me.

I wish with all my heart that I did not have The Huddle, but I *do* have them, and I seem to have

THE HUDDLE

almost reached the point of simply accepting the way that I am rather than continuing to nurture such hatred, anger and self pity about the fact that I am a voice hearer. It is not *wrong* to hear voices, just different, and perhaps acceptance of my lot would be a positive step. An analogy would be the diabetic who accepts their condition and the fact that they have to manage it, while at the same time not *liking* it and hoping that the cure is just around the corner. I know I would take the step of acceptance reluctantly and unhappily, yet all the while remembering what the apostle Paul said, "For I have learned, in whatsoever state I am, therein to be content." (Philippians 4:11) That's certainly a difficult one! Content whilst a hearer of their blasphemy? Content to be a hearer of their obscenities? Content to accept their constant mocking and humiliation of me? No! Definitely not! BUT – to accept that I have them does not mean accepting that they are acceptable! Simple that I *have* them and will strive to be content in my situation *despite* having to cope with them.

Rachel and I recently made a totally unplanned, unexpected and unwanted journey; a journey into the Church in Wales. Now then, considering my past dive into the occult, the fact that The Huddle are so against God, and my unfortunate and dangerous dealings with Reverend H, this is nothing short of a miracle! I swore that I would never set foot inside a church ever again, but I have done, we have done, and this is how it came about –

Janet Cooper

It was last September (it is now May 1997) when my daughter asked if she could join a church choir. Suddenly. Completely out of the blue.

"Mum. I want to sing in a church choir."

I was absolutely horrified, dead against it, and told her so, as gently as possible. I did not even understand where she had got the idea from as she'd never been to a church that had a choir. This was a perplexing mystery.

At the same time, I remembered, with some degree of fear, a verse of scripture that had been going round and round my head for several weeks, and I did not want to give thought to the possibility that this verse, plus Heather's request to join a church choir, were in any way connected. If they were, then that would point to some kind of divine intervention in my life and I'm rather good at denying that God would think me worthy of any of His attention. Or was this some dread Satanic trickery on the go?

No. It wasn't. How do I know that? Because Jesus shone a glimmer of light into the dungeon of my mind and exhorted me to go along with what was happening and what was about to happen. Also, the passage of time has indicated that everything that has happened since September last is positive, Godly, and certainly not of the devil! I have no doubt, however, even in the face of all the evidence that Reverend H, if he were to know about it, would think differently.

Anyway, where was I? Oh yes. Heather began pestering her father and I about this church choir business and we did everything we possibly could to put her off and get her to forget all about it. No

THE HUDDLE

go! She was utterly determined and increased her requests that we find a choir for her to join; and it *had* to be a church choir.

Frank finally crumbled under her persistence and reluctantly phoned the choirmaster of St. Woolos Cathedral to see if he would accept Heather as a chorister. He couldn't, as it was a 'boys only' choir, and I heaved a big sigh of relief and tried my best to comfort a distraught ten year old. But. This choirmaster had suggested that Frank should ring the choirmaster of St. John the Evangelist in Maindee, Newport, as this choir accepted both male and female voices. So, to cut a long story a bit shorter, the following Friday Heather attended her first choir practice and that very evening I found myself sewing nametags into her beautiful robes. I had such mixed feeling about it then. Fear, and pride, and not wanting to get interested or involved as it was a church she was singing in after all.

For the next three weeks Frank went to church twice every Sunday with Heather, who had taken to being a chorister like a proverbial duck takes to water. She loved it! I refused point blank even to go to church *once* and sit through a service in order to see her in her beloved choir. But she nagged and nagged me. And nagged me again. Then nagged me some more.

"Mum! Please! You've *got* to come! Please Mum?" And that verse of scripture kept repeating itself over and over again inside my head, and the more I tried to ignore it, the louder it became. I felt utterly compelled to listen to it. So, what was that verse?

"A little child shall lead them."

Then one Sunday I went, having crumbled under Heather's persistence and also feeling I should do this for my daughter, however difficult I might find it.

"I'll come, say, once a month Heth, in the evening when there are not so many people, okay?"

Yes, that was okay. But then the following week I went again! And again the following week, by which time I was totally shocked and horrified at the set up! Altars candles, people in robes, bowing to a metal cross.... It was Satanic! This was the stuff of covens! How can this be a Christian church? They had it all wrong……..

The choir and congregation chanted prayers and psalms like witches chanted spells and allegiance to the powers of darkness. Why the altar and its candles? Why were people bowing to this altar with its candles and metal cross? Who were they bowing to? Did they even know why they were doing it?

I was confused and horrified and The Huddle were having a field day about it. I was not able to see things in church as they really were. The white candles became black before my very eyes, the cross inverted itself and the robed clergy became Satanists holding out a cup of blood at the Eucharist from which all took a sip. Ugh!!

The Huddle settled themselves into a little red light in the corner of the church and mocked everything that went on during the services. I was in agony. It was difficult for me to concentrate and

THE HUDDLE

The Huddle were so tormentingly blasphemous that I decided, that third Sunday, that I would never go again. It was most definitely not for me and I wanted nothing more to do with it all thank-you very much! It was way too much to cope with on top of everything else and besides which, the man in the robes who seemed to be in charge, would probably 'do a Reverend' before long and ban me from attending his church if he ever found out that I was sat there with The Huddle and a head full of others! People like me should not be in church! (Reverend H, on 20th April 1990, *did* ban me from attending church! He would not allow me to return until I was completely delivered, that is, no longer hearing voices. Frank and the kids were 'allowed', even encouraged, to attend. But without me. How cruel is that? It had made me 'iller' than ever. The Huddle increased in volume and number and incessantly chanted the word 'banned' inside my head, leading to suicidal plans and attempts. My marriage and my family were very nearly torn apart. Reverend H told me repeatedly that God had told him to take this action.)

    Anyway, I somehow got through that last service probably by comforting myself that I would not inflict such torment on my brain ever again! I became totally rebellious, rebellious, refusing even to pick up the Book of Common Prayer. I would not sing any of the hymns and I kept my eyes wide open and my head up, defiantly, while everyone prayed. You crazy, deluded lot, I thought. You don't realise that all this is of the devil! Just look at that altar!! I was proud of my attitude.

Two days later, on a Tuesday night, Jan went to work. We came home the next morning and I went to bed to try and get a few hours sleep. I was very restless but eventually managed to doze off.

Rachel and I had a dream. We dreamt that we were quite alone in the church and we were arguing. About church. About other things too. I can't remember exactly. Then we began to fight, hitting out and trying to scratch each other. It was very vicious. Then Angel (Elinor?) came and stood before us and told us both to stop it and listen to her. We both became quiet and still, turning to face her.

"Join the choir!" She said. Rachel remained quiet but I started to argue with angel. Join the choir? Me? Us? Was that some sort of a sick joke? That was the last thing I wanted, nothing could have been further from my mind, and I never wanted to set foot in that church ever again, never mind sing in their flaming choir! No way! I can't and I won't and that's final!!!

"You must both join the choir. Both of you." Said Angel, quietly but with authority.

No way, I thought again. I can't. The Huddle won't let me.....

"Join the choir!" Angel repeated.

It's impossible, I told her. What about Easter? What about Christmas? Can you *imagine* what The Huddle would be like with Rachel and I singing in a *church* choir? I WILL NOT!!!!!

"Join the choir." Angel persisted.

I awoke following this disturbing dream. "Bitch is awake!" Rachel immediately asked me what I was going to do about Angel's 'join the choir.' I replied

THE HUDDLE

that it was only a stupid dream and I wasn't going to do *anything* about it! Rachel was quiet then, unusually, and passed no comment. 'A little child shall lead them'. I shook my head to try and get those words, and the stupid dream, out of my mind.

Hours later Heather came home from school, had some tea, and then, right out of the blue again, suddenly said to me,

"Mum, you ought to join the choir." I said a very definite no thank-you!

"Aw, come on Mum! Join the choir and come with me, I'll look after you, I'll help you. Why not, Mum?" No. Definitely not, Heth.

"Well, you *should* join the choir you know, Mum!" I was starting to get pretty annoyed by then and so Heather beat a hasty retreat outside to play with a friend.

I sat down at the dining table, troubled and unsettled, waiting for Frank to arrive home from work. It was as I sat there alone (well, you know what I mean!) that I made a sudden decision, and as soon as I had made it I was flooded with a glorious, warm sense of relief and certainty that I was about to do the right thing. In fact, I felt very, very, *very* good about it! I was going to join the choir!!

Two days later I attended my first choir practice and absolutely love it from the words go! I loved the people, the music, the singing, the church, the everything! There were no spare robes for me so I would not be able to sing in church with them for a while, so I would just attend the practices for a few weeks. Good, I thought, that would give me a chance to really settle in and get used to the idea.

However, two days after that, on Sunday, I was told that there *were* robes for me after all, and so it has happened that since then I have 'robed up' twice every Sunday and sung to Jesus in a holy place! The ecstasy of doing that! The agony of The Huddle's response to it.

Heather has actually taken me and Rachel by the hand and led us into the vestry week after week. 'A little child shall lead them.' She has been such a help and has persisted in her encouragement and belief that I *must* continue to sing thus. One sadness is that her brother does not want to give church a try at the moment. We understand and we don't push him. Jesus is everywhere.

I wrote and told Elinor (I call her that now) that I had joined a choir and she expressed her delight next time I saw her. I had half expected her to be horrified and surprised but she, too, felt very, very good about it and also understood my difficulties over such an about turn.

I'd had, only a few weeks before, another encounter with an evil comforter, initiated by myself, and Elinor had been so worried about me that one Saturday afternoon she had decided to meet with a friend to pray about me. We later met and found out that the time Elinor had decided to pray was the time I experienced a sudden lifting of the terrible depression I had fallen into following the invocation of this wretched evil comforter. Elinor had prayed with her friend then paid me an extra, unexpected visit the following Monday.

I had not wanted her to come because, in the company of my evil comforter, I had planned for

THE HUDDLE

Jan to work my usual Tuesday night, but instead of coming straight home I would travel to the Brecon Beacons with a bottle of tablets and a can of coke. I would be dead before anyone found me. But along came Elinor, seeming to know what I was planning, afraid that I would carry it out, and wanting to speak very seriously to me. I was maybe quite rude and nasty to her; I can't remember. She asked how I felt about this extra visit of hers and I merely shrugged my shoulders. She had come to stop me killing myself and I was absolutely bloody furious about it!!

Obviously, I did not kill myself that Wednesday. Instead, I decided that I would still go to the Brecon Beacons and, as I had done before, I would leave my evil comforter there. Again! But how wonderful Jesus is! For no sooner had I made my decision to be rid of this evil thing, Jesus spoke to me.

"It is done!"

And I knew instantly that my evil comforter had left me. The burden of having to kill myself was lifted from me so gently, and Jesus had not required me to make any great efforts or travel any great distance. How opposite He is to Satan!

I remembered how I'd felt forced and pushed half way up Caerphilly mountain in the midst of a howling gale and lashing rain in order to invoke that evil comforter. What ridiculous things Satan pushes you to do! How depressed and desperate I must have felt to go along with him! How gentle, kind and understanding Jesus is in comparison!

But now here I was in a church choir and Elinor was so pleased for me. And for Rachel. Rachel and I had come closer together in a most wonderful and unexpected way. God's way? We now help each other; we sympathise over our separate difficulties. Rachel does the bits I can't do, like taking the bread and wine, and walking down the aisle in the processionals at the beginning and ending of services. I sort out our music, find the right hymns and psalms, and chat to the other choristers as best I can. We do the singing together. We wear a red cassock and a beautiful white surplice.

Whilst I tend to fret and worry and question the need for all this dressing up, Rachel loves it, and there is for both of us an awestruck sense of privilege in being clothed in white and allowed to be in a church singing to Jesus! It is beautiful and humbling. It is also very difficult for us. We'll keep at it for we know that somehow it's worth the effort.

Elinor listened intently to Rachel and I as we told her about our difficulties with attending church. Seeing the candles as black, the upside down cross, the Huddle, Rachel's voices, which include that of Reverend H. He, I know, is particularly distressing for her. We both of us also fear being banned again. (Who the hell gets banned from a church of all places??) We feel unwanted and unsafe on an earthly level and are extremely nervous of the vicar and the other clergy. It was all so strange, so scary, and yet so very wonderful.

Elinor then had an idea, following which she was able to arrange for me to go with her to meet with the Christian author, Una Kroll. Una is one of life's lovely people, and her prayers and Godly wisdom helped Rachel and I in many ways. She told me to listen to Rachel. I have done, and, amazingly, have come to love her. I call her, affectionately, my little nun in a cell!

THE HUDDLE

Following our visit to Una, Elinor and I went to a pretty little café for something to eat and a cup of tea before the journey home. It was there, over my toasted teacake and Elinor's strawberry gateau, that Dr. Kapp, the psychiatrist who told me she was also my friend, became Elinor, my friend who also happened to be a psychiatrist. As we sat and talked, it just happened. I no longer felt that I needed to keep her at some safe distance and it was wonderful to feel I had a real friend at last. Also scary. Would it last? I doubted it, knowing my luck!

So things were changing. For so long I hadn't been able to want to feel better and bother to stay alive, yet I did agree to visit somebody who might be able to help me, so dared to assume that things really were changing for the better. But were they? Time would tell.

I feel as if I am making a mess of this last bit of my book. Is it too rambling and discursive and the usual boring rubbish? No matter. My book. I can say what I like. The Huddle are in the desk lamp as usual and I am now frowning as I type through transparent worms. Ugh............. Stop a while.......

Dreams still come every night. Now they are dreams about the Huddle battering the choir to death, but however much they batter us, we still sing! They cannot stop us singing! How wonderful!

In other dreams bad things are happening in church. Rachel is screaming, my robes are torn off me, the communion wine becomes blood, Satan snakes around the candles and there is no light.......

Janet Cooper

How I am, we are, is agony and it is ecstasy. From darkness to light. From hate to love. From the coven to the choir stalls. From Satan to Jesus. From pain to healing. From death into life………?

The Huddle are demonic, evil and against God. My answer seems to lie in struggling to go in a direction opposite to them. That is, to follow the teachings of Christ. He *must* be my way, my truth, my light and my life. In Him is no darkness. The ugliness of The Huddle shall be cancelled out by His beauty, their cruelty by His gentleness, their hatred by His love.

Finally, finally, finally…..

May God be in this head, now and for evermore?
Then, and only ever then…….
AMEN!

THE HUDDLE

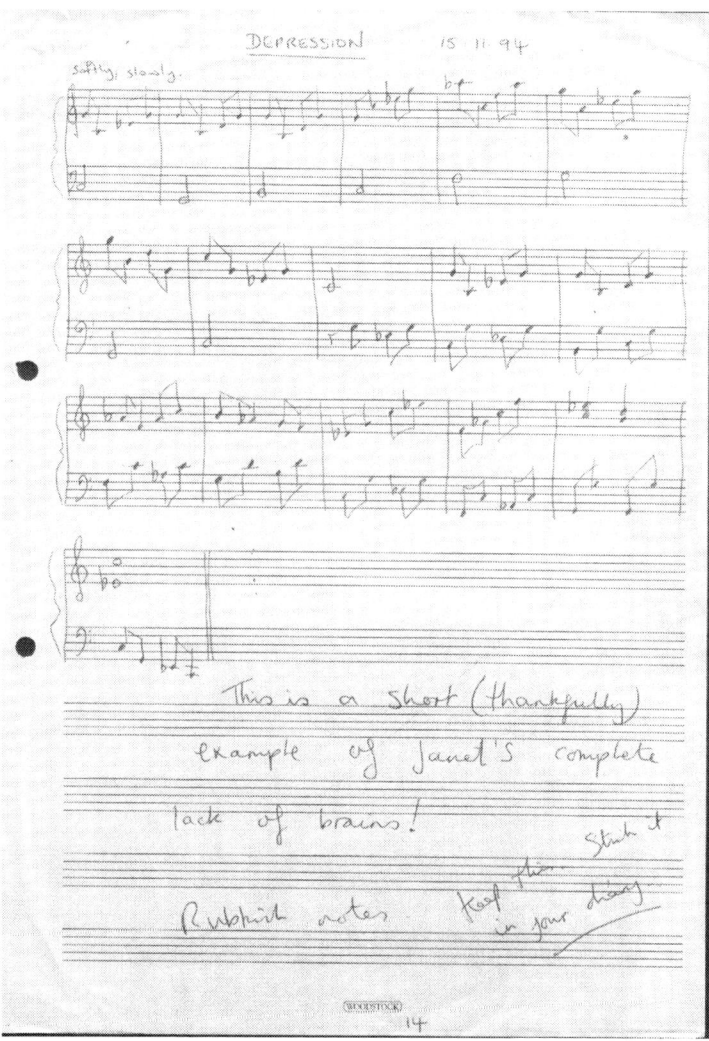

Janet Cooper

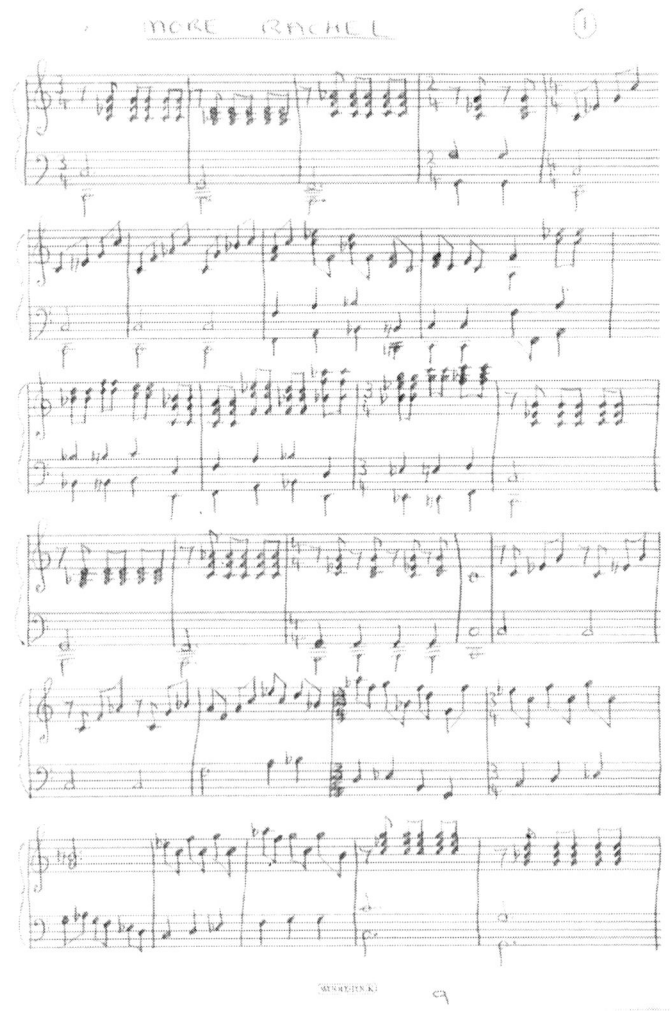

THE HUDDLE

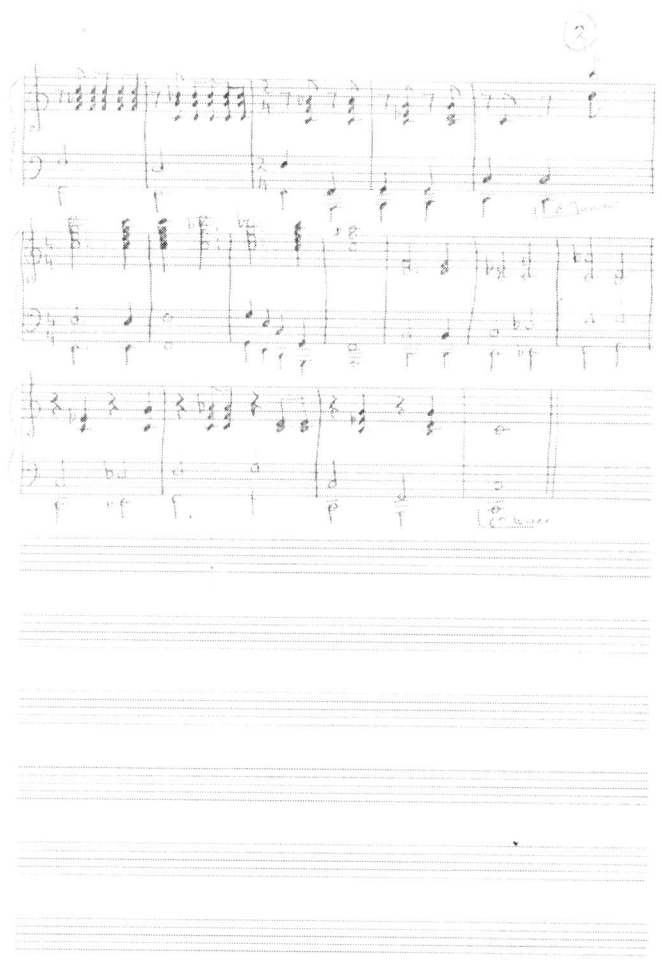

Janet Cooper

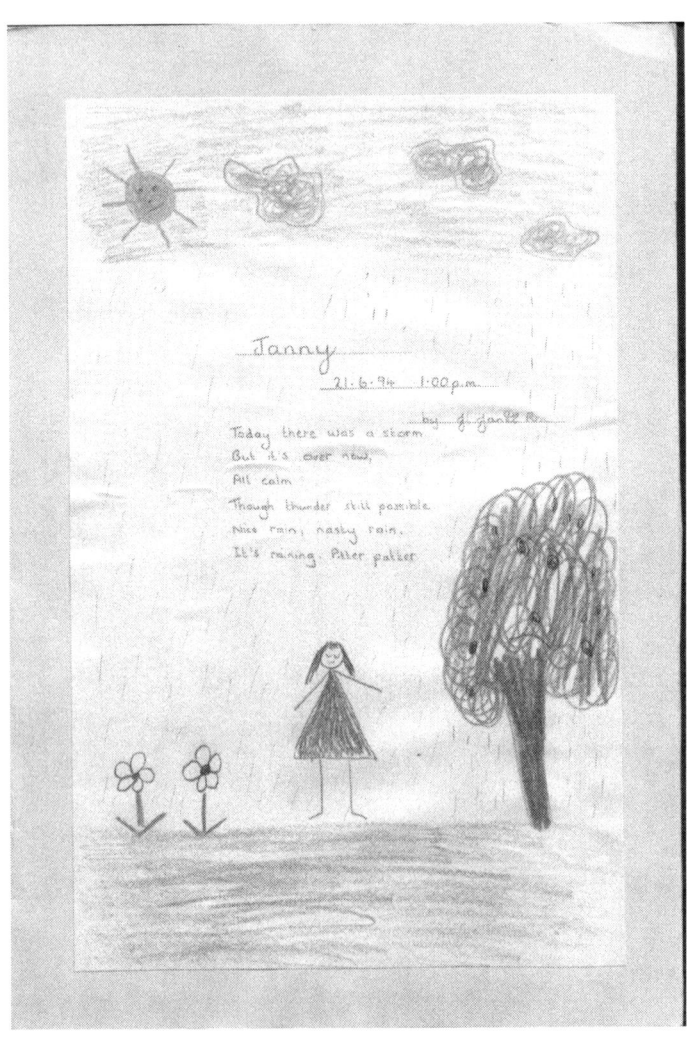

THE HUDDLE

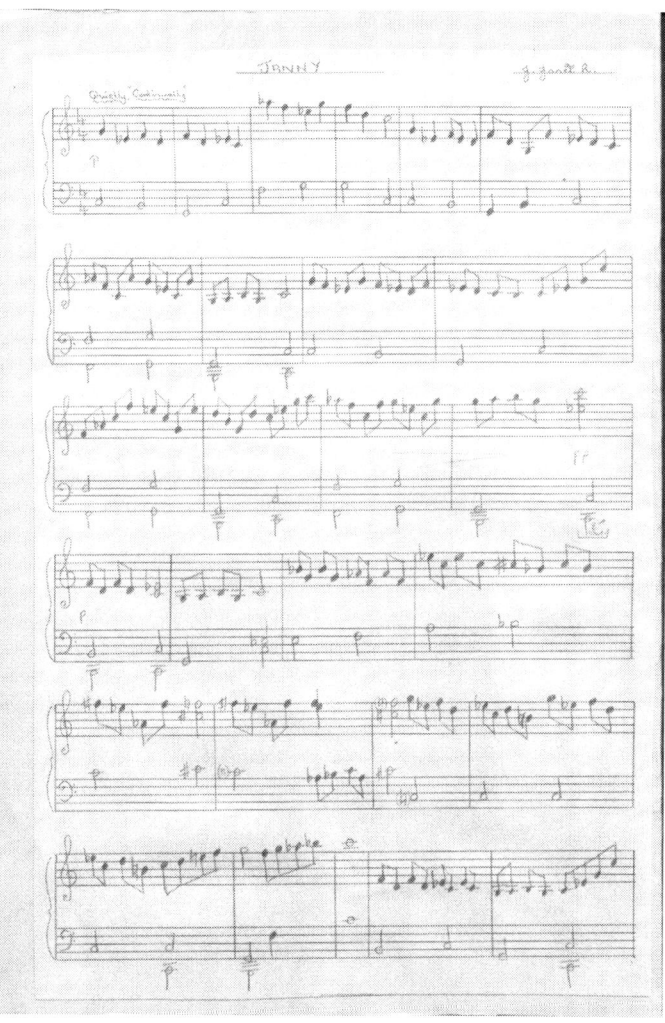

Janet Cooper

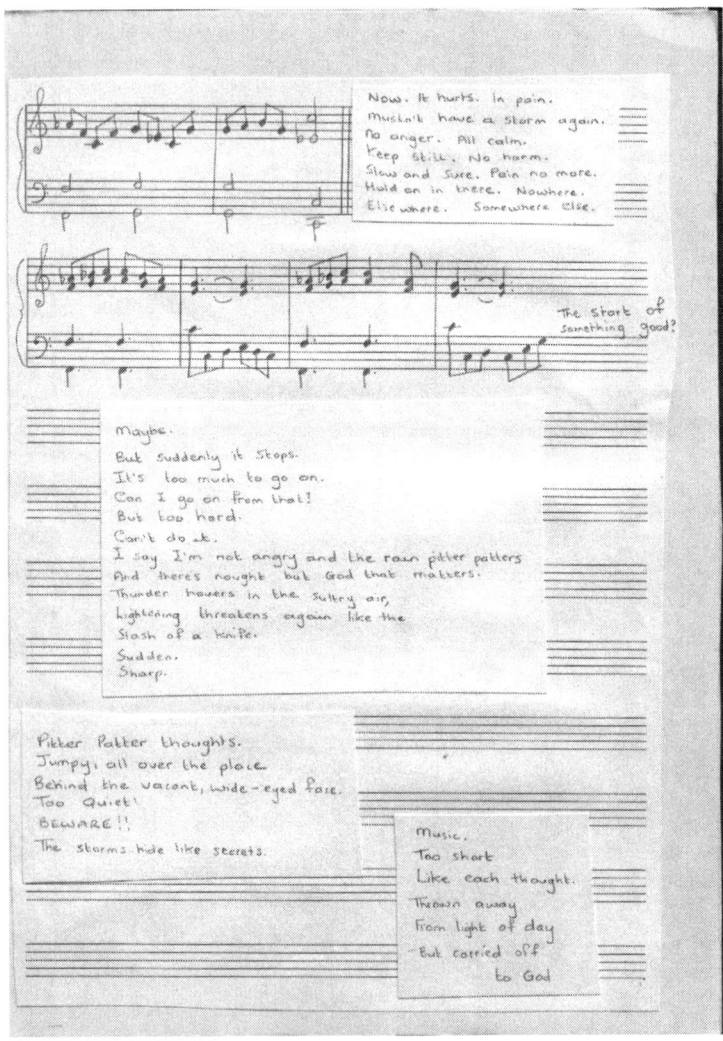

THE HUDDLE

Printed in the United Kingdom by
Lightning Source UK Ltd., Milton Keynes
142584UK00001B/5/P